The Ultimate Guide to Anal Sex for Women

by Tristan Taormino

Illustrated by Fish

CLEIS
PRESS

Published in the United States by Cleis Press Inc., P.O. Box 14684, San Francisco, California 94114.

Printed in the United States.
Cover and text design: Karen Huff
Logo art: Juana Alicia
First Edition.
10 9 8 7 6 5 4 3 2

Illustrations copyright © 1998 by Fish.

for Felice,

whose heart and soul

are in here

Acknowledgments

There are so many people whom I'd like to thank for their contributions to this project.

To Felice Newman and Frédérique Delacoste, for their time, devotion, and gracious understanding of an insanely hectic schedule. Special thanks to Felice, to whom this book is dedicated, for going beyond the call—and even farther than that.

To Susie Bright, Pat Califia, everyone at Good Vibrations, Nina Hartley, Bert Herrman, Jack Morin, Carol Queen, Anne Semans, and Cathy Winks for their extraordinary, groundbreaking work.

To Robert Morgan for unbelievable generosity and kindness.

To Tammy Fortin at Aardvark Books, The New York Public Library, Amazon.com, the Society for Human Sexuality, and San Francisco Sex Information for research assistance.

To Nancy Bereano of Firebrand Books, Joan Nestle, Greg Constante of Alyson Publications, Pat Califia, and Sarah Miller for permission to reprint their work.

To Russ Kick, Bill Brent, and The Black Book for tremendous help with the resource guide.

To Karen Green, Don Spargo, Jr., and Rosana Francescato for insightful editorial advice.

To Tom Bates for making a whole lot possible. To Chip Rowe for being The Man.

To Thia "Fish" Jennings for her wit, her understanding, and her brilliant illustrations.

To everyone who responded to my survey for being so generous and sharing intimate details of their lives.

To Kate Bornstein, Bree Coven, Morgan Dunbar, Gerry Gomez Pearlberg, Mario Grillo, Colin Hall, Ron Lieber, Dan Mitchell, Audrey Prins-Patt, Janet Schomer, and D. Travers Scott for their friendship, love, and support.

To Karen Green for too much to even name.

To Winston Wilde for being my daddy.

To my mother, Judith Pynchon, for always supporting me.

And, finally, to my dogs, Reggie Love and Jordan Love, who are my constant companions during late-night research, reading, writing, and revisions.

Contents

Introduction • 1

Confessions of a Backdoor Betty:
Why I Love Anal Sex and Why I Wrote This Book

1

10 Myths About Anal Sex • 13

Myth #1: Anal sex is unnatural and immoral.
Myth #2: Only sluts, perverts, and weirdos have anal sex.
Myth #3: The anus and rectum were never meant to be
    eroticized.
Myth #4: Anal sex is dirty and messy.
Myth #5: Only homosexual men have anal sex.
Myth #6: Straight men who like anal sex are really gay.
Myth #7: Anal sex is always painful for the person on the
    receiving end.
Myth #8: Women don't enjoy receiving anal sex; they do it
    just to please their partners.
Myth #9: Anal sex is the easiest way to get AIDS.
Myth #10: Anal sex is naughty.

2

Our Asses, Ourselves • 21

A Brief Anatomy Lesson
    The Anus, Anal Sphincters, and PC Muscles
    Exercising Your Pelvic and PC Muscles
    The Anal Canal and the Rectum
Basic Preparations
    Short, Smooth Nails
    Clean Tools
    Clean Butt and Empty Bowels
    Relaxation
    Safety First

3   **Beyond Our Bodies: Emotional and Psychological Aspects of Anal Eroticism • 39**

Desire
Communication
Fear
Expectations, Needs, and Fantasies
Patience
Presence
Trust and Power

4   **Tools of the Trade • 49**

Latex
Lubricants
Butt Plugs
Vibrators
Dildos
Anal Beads
Tips

5   **Shaving and Enemas: Spring Cleaning and Then Some • 67**

Enemas
    Bulb Syringe Enemas
    Enema Bag/Hot Water Bottle Enemas
    Shower Attachment Enemas
    General Tips for a Safe Enema
The Barber and the Back Door: Shaving the Anal Area

6   **Doing It for Yourself: Masturbation and Anal Eroticism • 75**

7   **Let Your Tongue Do the Walking • 81**

Analingus
Analingus and Safer Sex

8   **Anal Penetration • 86**

Insertive Anal Penetration
Receptive Anal Penetration
For Both Partners
Positions for Anal Penetration

9   **Anal Fisting • 102**

Myths About Anal Fisting
Anal Fisting and Safer Sex
Anal Fisting: The How-To's

10   **S/M and Genderplay • 112**

S/M and Anal Sex
Genderplay and Anal Sex

11   **Anal Health • 120**

Taking Care of Your Ass
Anal Ailments
Anal Sex and STDs
HIV and AIDS

12   **The Ultimate Frontier • 130**

Resources • 133

Books
Publications
Shopping Guide
Sex Information Resources
World Wide Web Resources

Index • 145
About the Author • 153
About the Illustrator • 153

Illustrations

1. Female Anatomy / Page 22
2. Anorectal Anatomy / Page 27
3. Male Anatomy / Page 29
4. Anal Toys / Page 50
5. Female Condom / Page 52
6. Putting on a Condom / Page 54
7. Enema Equipment / Page 68
8. Making a Dental Dam / Page 85
9. Missionary / Page 95
10. On Top / Page 97
11. Doggie-Style / Page 99
12. Spooning / Page 100

Introduction

**Confessions of a Backdoor Betty:
Why I Love Anal Sex
and Why I Wrote This Book**

Confessions

Yes, I admit it—I love anal sex. The first time someone put a finger in my butt, I almost went crazy from the pleasure. The sensations I experienced were so intense, incredible, and heavenly that it was mind-blowing. I felt high from the experience, and I couldn't wait to do it again. The first time I put my finger in someone else's butt, the results were just as fabulous—I felt entrusted with my partner's deepest vulnerabilities, in awe of the ecstatic pleasure I could give. Then came more fingers, tongues, vibrators, small dildos, bigger dildos, butt plugs, a penis, bigger butt plugs, even an entire small hand.

Each time I could take a little more and give a little more, I felt more sexually alive and powerful. As I incorporated anal eroticism into my sex life, my sex life became better and better. The sex got hotter, my partners extra adventurous, my orgasms fierce and explosive. The physical sensations were undeniably some of the best I'd ever felt in my life. I confess too that beyond the deep body gratification, the naughtiness of it all really turned me on. Even my most kinky, sexually liberated friends weren't doing *this*—or if they were, they never talked about it (and I knew the intimate details of everything else they were doing in bed). Only sexually voracious gay men fucked each other's asses with abandon the way I was. Neither my partners nor I identified as gay men, so what did we think we were doing?

Too Many Myths

Growing up in this culture, it is nearly impossible to escape the taboo of anal sexuality and all the myths surrounding it. From an early age, we are taught that our assholes are private, dirty, and shouldn't be touched in a sexual way. Whether we learn about the birds and the bees from popular books or in sex education class, the anus is rarely mentioned, unless to say it's behind our genitals. As I grew up, I heard "fag jokes" about men who "do each other in the butt"; these men were derided for their practice of anal sex. If we do hear about people other than gay men having sex, they are usually labeled "kinky" or "perverted," and the sex is clearly considered abnormal. When anal sex is acknowledged as an erotic preference in sex research and popular advice columns, it is portrayed as a fantasy of straight men whose women partners endure pain in order to please. There are rarely representations of women who enjoy anal sex with either men or women. Most recently, anal sex has been linked to the AIDS virus and represented as dangerous and even deadly.

I became sexually active in the eighties, just at the beginning of the AIDS crisis; by the time I became more sexually literate and experienced and discovered the pleasures of anal sex, AIDS had become epidemic. Because gay men were becoming infected in alarming numbers, they became designated *the* high-risk group. According to the majority of safer sex guidelines at the time, anal sex was how you got AIDS. And I was having anal sex. It's scary when major medical institutions tell you that one of your favorite things to do in the world is no longer just naughty, but actually life-threatening.

The progress made in the sexually liberated 1970s and the decadent 1980s, which contributed to a wider acceptance of many sexual practices previously considered taboo (including anal sex), was squelched by AIDS phobia in the 1990s. For example, in the first edition of the very popular *The Joy of Sex*, published in 1972, Dr. Alex Comfort writes:

> This [anal intercourse] is something which nearly every couple tries once. A few stay with it usually because the woman finds that it gives her intenser feelings than the normal route and is pleasurably tight for the man.[1]

However, in *The New Joy of Sex: A Gourmet Guide to Lovemaking for the Nineties*, Comfort describes the rectum as "a canal primarily engineered for other purposes." He dismisses the practice of anal sex because of the risks associated with HIV infection: "In the light of present knowledge, this is best avoided altogether."[2]

When the fear of AIDS first became widespread, much of the so-called safer sex guidelines were rife with misinformation. The same institutions releasing propaganda about safer sex claimed that heterosexuals and lesbians weren't at risk. Then heterosexuals and lesbians started getting sick. Members of the gay community and AIDS activists realized that the key to saving lives was having correct information and making it widely available. The problem is that myths and misinformation about anal sex are rampant in our society, while accurate statistics, facts, personal experiential accounts, and healthy, positive representations are nearly impossible to find. Soon, activists realized that they had to start producing their own information.

The Truth About Girls and Boys

Of the little that has been written about anal eroticism, much has been by and for men who have anal sex with other men. In fact, in spite of the cultural taboo and largely because of AIDS, many members of the gay community have openly acknowledged that gay men have anal sex. In general, gay men seem to embrace anal sexuality and discuss it more honestly than others. In the wake of the AIDS epidemic and its devastating effects on the gay male community, exploration of the practice and risks of anal sex has become a way to save lives. Yet, because discussions, informative workshops, and literature tend to be community-based, people outside the community don't always have access to them.

This book is written primarily for women who want to learn more about anal sex and health and to explore insertive and receptive anal pleasure with women, men, and transgender people. My work focuses on the particular psychological, emotional, physical, and health-related issues that women face. Although the book concentrates on the experiences of women, many of the guidelines and generalizations about anal sex apply to everyone, regardless of gender.

"I'd Like Another, Please, Sir"

It is surprising to me that only one book exists that is devoted solely to anal eroticism: *Anal Pleasure and Health* by Jack Morin. While it is an incredibly ground-breaking, informative, and insightful work, it seems odd that it is the only one in a field populated by so much selection and variety. I recently decided to investigate just what sex books are being sold in America's book-stores. As my test site, I chose a well-known national chain bookstore in a fairly conservative neighborhood of Manhattan. As I perused the shelves of the "Sexuality" section, I found an extensive selection. The majority of the books were devoted to improving the sexual aware-ness and the sex lives of readers—they discussed how to have hot sex, better sex, orgasmic sex, more sex, and safer sex. There were books by sex therapists, sexologists, sex researchers, sex workers, sex advisors, and other sex-uality specialists. There were even a half-dozen titles dedicated to fairly alternative sexual practices, such as sadomasochism (S/M), dominance and submission, pain and pleasure, and bondage and discipline. Obviously, there is a significant market for sex books. This is due in part to our society's obsession with sex and sexuality, but it also reflects the importance of sex in our lives. People are hungry for information, ideas, and advice on all aspects of sexuality.

Among the thousands of books about sex currently in print, many are quite focused and specialized, covering such topics as solo sex, oral sex, vibrator sex, sex after fifty, fantasy sex, lesbian sex, phone sex, role-playing sex, gay sex, tantric sex, healing sex, transgender sex, cyber-sex, leather sex, kinky sex. There are also titles devoted to erotic massage, foreplay, romance, cross-dressing, monogamy, and nonmonogamy. And yet among the sea of sex volumes, there is only one about anal sex.

Anal Pleasure Stuck in the Margins

In general self-help sex manuals and other books that claim to cover the full spectrum of sexual practices, anal sex usually receives a mere few pages or a couple of sentences—if it is not left out altogether. In popular titles like Dr. Ruth Westheimer's *Sex for Dummies*™ and *Sex in America: A Definitive Survey*, there is only brief information about anal eroticism and health. The coverage of anal sexuality pales in comparison to thoughtful, thorough, and informative sections on just about every other kind of sexuality; in addition, the information presented is often negative, mis-informed, outdated, and even incorrect. So, while these volumes are described as "complete," "definitive," and "comprehensive," those of us searching for information on anal pleasure are often left wondering why it's missing.

Media Representations M.I.A.

If anal sex is in the margins of written works, it's off the map in other media. When was the last time you saw a positive representation of anal eroticism in a film? When was the last time someone mentioned anal sex on televi-sion? In a mainstream magazine? When I asked a group of women where they had seen representations of anal sex, the responses included:

- *Anal Pleasure and Health*, by Jack Morin (the only book of its kind)
- *Try* (a novel) and other works by Dennis Cooper
- *Trust* (a guide to handballing, or anal fisting), by Bert Herrman
- The original edition of *The Joy of Sex*
- Lesbian erotica
- *The Story of O* (classic erotic S/M novel), by Pauline Réage
- *The Lesbian S/M Safety Manual*, edited by Pat Califia
- *Sapphistry : The Book of Lesbian Sexuality*, by Pat Califia

- The Good Vibrations mail-order catalog
- Gay male erotic magazines and videos
- Chester Mainard's anal massage video
- Porn videos
- Leather-S/M community workshops

One respondent said: "From my perspective, I think there's mostly been a dearth of information, a loud silence, about women's—especially heterosexual women's—anal desires."

Because American media is consumed with sex and sexuality, many of the images we see on a daily basis—from soap operas and beer commercials to music videos and magazine ads—are saturated with sex. However, there is a great big void when it comes to anal sex.

Where Do Women Get Information About Anal Sex?

Women have many sources for information about sexual health and practices: family doctors, gynecologists, other health care professionals, therapists, parents, siblings, and friends. However, these sources generally don't provide information about anal health and sexuality. When was the last time you talked to one of these people about anal sex? While we may talk to any number of people about sexual health, STDs, birth control, and safer sex, most women don't feel comfortable discussing anal sexuality, and most experts don't bring up the subject. Even when I've been thoroughly quizzed on my sexual practices during a gynecological exam, the subject of anal sex and health has never come up.

Who Am I?

As you've probably noticed, no titles or initials appear before or after my name—no M.D., Ph.D., M.A., C.S.W., or M.S.W. I am not a doctor, psychiatrist, psychotherapist, or sex therapist, although I have studied the work of many people who are. As I explained before, I am less of an anal expert than an ass aficionado and student. I have combed sex self-help books, sex research studies, sex surveys, sex advice columns and books, health manuals, safer sex guidelines, and various erotic materials for information on anal sexuality. I've tried to learn as much as I can about anal anatomy, health, and sexuality and have relied on other more qualified individuals for areas outside my own knowledge and experience. I have attempted to write about the subject in a form and language that everyone can understand.

What Anal Sex Is and What It Isn't

While there has been a great deal of silence and little research about anal sex, the mythology, practices, and representations of anal sex have a complex history. One could write an entire book analyzing the anal taboo in American society; the myths about anal eroticism could be the central theme of another book. And don't forget these worthwhile topics: the etymology of anal sex, theoretical and critical discourses about anal sex and society, and the psychology and psychoanalytic history of anal sex. Some impressive work has been done in these areas, and more work is certainly needed. I give an overview of the anal taboo and related myths in chapter 1, and throughout the book I refer to any number of these larger historical and theoretical issues as they relate to anal sex. They have informed my own thinking about anal sexuality. However, this book is meant to be not a theoretical work but a hands-on, useful, and practical resource for people interested in exploring anal sexuality.

Survey Says

In order to incorporate the experiences, attitudes, feelings, and perspectives of other women, I conducted a small, confidential, written survey of women who have had anal sex with women, men, or transgendered people. I sent a survey containing thirty-six questions to colleagues and contacts and encouraged them to pass it on to others. I took a qualitative approach over a quantitative one, as I was more interested in the details of people's feelings and experiences than in compiling statistics. I asked respondents questions about a variety of matters: their first encounters with anal eroticism; anal activities they've experienced; giving and receiving anal pleasure; anal erotic likes and dislikes; anal sex positions; toys used for anal stimulation and penetration; desires, fantasies, and fears associated with anal sex; gender play, role-playing, and S/M; STDs, HIV, and AIDS; sources for information about anal sexuality; and media representations of anal sex. I have incorporated excerpts from the questionnaires throughout the book (set off in italics) in order to illustrate important points and to give readers a glimpse of some real-life opinions, feelings, and experiences other than my own. The quotes are meant to capture the voices of individuals and what they have to say about anal eroticism; they are not meant to represent norms, values, and beliefs among women in general.

A Road Map

First, a word about terminology. I have tried to be as explicit and specific as possible in this book. When I use the term *anal sex,* I mean it to encompass *all* forms of anal eroticism, including manual stimulation, oral stimulation, and anal penetration of all kinds.

The first chapter explores myths and facts about anal sex. The anal taboo and anal sex myths are both prevalent and well-rooted in American society. These myths, based on fear more than fact, often prevent people from voicing their anal desires and acting on those desires. The first chapter is a good place to begin exploring these myths more closely. If we challenge the deeply ingrained notions behind them and discover how they have affected our own attitudes about the anus and its erotic potential, we can begin to replace those myths with truths. In addition, you may find the facts useful for communicating about anal sex and dispelling any misinformation you or your partner may have.

In the second chapter, I provide a brief anatomy lesson, covering related muscles and body parts, and encourage you to get better aquainted with your anus. In addition, I discuss some basics—hygiene, relaxation, safety—you should know about before beginning anal exploration of any kind to ensure that you're taking good care of your body.

In chapter 3, I discuss some of the ways we can take care of ourselves emotionally and psychologically, covering topics like desire, communication, fear, and patience. In addition, I explore some of the issues that may come up during anal sex with a partner, including fantasy, power dynamics, and trust.

Chapter 4 includes a discussion of latex condoms, gloves, and dental dams as well as different kinds of lubricants. There is a guide to the various tools you can use to enhance anal pleasure, including butt plugs, vibrators, dildos, and anal beads, and some hints about how to assess the safety of any other tool you're thinking of using for anal sex.

You may feel inclined to skip right away to chapters 5–10, but be patient; it's important to read the preceding chapters first to ensure you are well prepared for anal sex. Chapters 5–10 cover the ins and outs of anal masturbation, analingus (also called rimming), insertive anal penetration, and receptive anal penetration, as well as other activities, including enemas (or anal douching), shaving the anal area, anal fisting (inserting a hand in someone's rectum), S/M and anal play, and gender play.

Chapter 11 is an important one for everyone to read. It covers general anal health and how to maintain a healthy, happy anus. In addition, I discuss several common sexually transmitted diseases (STDs), how they are transmitted, general symptoms and treatments, HIV, AIDS, and safer sex practices. The information about various diseases is written specifically as it relates to anal sexuality.

Throughout the book, I have included brief excerpts from erotic literature and quotes from popular books and magazines. My research references recent, well-known sex studies and books. I hope these brief erotic passages will encourage you to enact your own anal fantasies and enjoy the full range of anal eroticism. I have also included exercises designed to help you explore and practice some of the topics discussed. At the end of the book, I have included a resource guide, with selected books and other sources for people who want to learn more about anal sex.

It is time for anal sex to come out of our closets. The more dialogue and information we initiate, the more we can all have our sexual desires and practices validated and can really begin to enhance our sex lives with ideas, techniques, and facts about anal sex. I want this book to empower women with knowledge about our bodies and sexualities. I want women to have safe and pleasurable anal sex with ourselves and our partners. And, while the cover touts this book as the "Ultimate Guide," I don't consider it the final word by any means. I hope it is just the beginning—the beginning of more discussion, more research, more investigation, and more exploration of the world of anal sexuality.

I hope beginners, fans, and experts alike will use and enjoy this book to help fulfill, improve, and enhance their explorations of anal sex. I know that the moment I discovered anal eroticism and shared it with a lover was a huge turning point in my erotic life. And it still drives me crazy after all this time.

Tristan Taormino
New York City
September 1997

NOTES
1. Alex Comfort, *The Joy of Sex: A Gourmet Guide to Lovemaking* (New York: Crown Publishers, 1972), 126.

2. Alex Comfort, *The New Joy of Sex: A Gourmet Guide to Lovemaking for the Nineties* (New York: Crown Publishers, 1991), 244.

3. Jack Morin, Leo Bersani, and Cindy Patton, among other scholars, have written some resourceful theoretical work about anal sexuality. See Resources at the end of this book for more information.

10 Myths About Anal Sex

Myth #1: Anal sex is unnatural and immoral.

TRUTH: Students of sociology and social change are aware of the axiom that today's deviance may well be tomorrow's norm. The present widespread approval of the practice of masturbation and oral sex is an example of a deviance of yesteryear that has changed into a norm. The definitions of what is or what isn't deviant behavior are established by various legitimate institutions, the most important being government and religion.[1]

The anal sex taboo is well established in American culture. Prevalent in religious, legal, medical, and scientific institutions, the taboo is clearly manifested in information about health and sexuality. The myths that follow will be familiar to most people, and they both inform and reinforce the anal sex taboo. Taboos usually defy logic, science, and experience; they generally have more to do with misinformation, fear, and a desire to maintain the status quo. In the case of anal sex, the taboo mirrors some fundamental elements of our society. For example, anal sex being considered dirty is linked with the cultural obsession with hygiene and cleanliness; the perceived connection between anal sex and gay men reflects deep-seated societal homophobia. Both so-called facts prevent people from experiencing anal pleasure.

In *Anal Pleasure and Health*, Jack Morin traces the religious roots of the anal sex taboo:

> In the Judeo-Christian tradition, the taboo against anal intercourse is seen as coming from God. In the Old Testament story, God completely destroys the city of Sodom, presumably as punishment for rampant sodomy among its people. Many scholars now believe that the punishment was for Sodom's violation of hospitality rules, and had little, if anything, to do with sex. The sodomy interpretation, however, is still one generally accepted. Among believers, condemnation of anal sex is not based on any discernible principle except the desire to avoid the wrath of God.[2]

Today, the people and institutions invested in maintaining that anal sex is unnatural and immoral are often the same folks who support antigay legislation, banning sex education in schools, and sodomy laws, which make it illegal to have any kind of sex other than procreative, heterosexual vaginal intercourse.

Myth #2: Only sluts, perverts, and weirdos have anal sex.

TRUTH: Anal sex is practiced and enjoyed by women, men, and transgender people of all kinds, from the perky girl next door to the daring dominatrix in the dungeon. In fact, in today's sex surveys and self-help books, the sections on "kinky" or "deviant" sex practices—including bondage, cross-dressing, S/M, golden showers, and group sex—do not usually include anal sex. Anal sex is more often categorized with vaginal intercourse and oral sex.[3] The notion that anal sex is kinky, abnormal, or perverted is based on the assumption that only a few specific kinds of sex—usually heterosexual, procreative, penis-vagina intercourse—are natural, normal, and conventional.

My BEST FRIEND, Jane, called me a few weeks ago. "I beat you," she said.

"You beat me? You have a job, your boyfriend went to Princeton, and you live in a major city. I'm sporadically employed in a town with, like, one off-ramp, and my boyfriend went to a minor Midwestern university and thinks deodorant is bourgeois. The only thing I have on you is that I'm a bigger slut."

"That," she said, "is precisely how I beat you."

"You had anal sex."

"Bingo."

My heart sank. "You must be very pleased with yourself."

"Honey, you have no idea."

—SARAH MILLER

Myth #3: The anus and rectum were never meant to be eroticized.

TRUTH: The anus and rectum are full of sensitive, responsive nerve endings, and the stimulation of these nerve endings and penetration of the rectum can be intensely pleasurable—and orgasmic—for both men and women. Furthermore, women's G-spots and perineums can be stimulated during anal sex, and men may experience stimulation of the bulb of the penis and the prostate gland through anal penetration. *The New Good Vibrations Guide to Sex* reminds us that "the anus is rich in nerve endings and participates with our genitals in the engorgement, muscular tension and contractions of sexual arousal and orgasm." [4]

Myth #4: Anal sex is dirty and messy.

TRUTH: As long as you practice standard hygiene, anal sex is no more messy than any other kind of sex. Feces are stored in the bowel and pass through the rectum and anal canal during a bowel movement. Normally, there is only a very small amount of fecal matter in the anal canal and rectum. Some people like to take a shower or bath before sex to clean the anal area, but no other extraordinary measures are necessary for anal sex. Some people have an enema before anal sex, but again, that is not necessary. (Read more about cleaning in chapter 2 and enemas in chapter 5).

Myth #5: Only homosexual men have anal sex.

TRUTH: People of all sexual orientations and partners of all genders have anal sex. While it's true that many gay men do have anal sex, the actual statistics reveal a much smaller percentage than is widely believed: 50–60 percent have tried it and fewer than 30 percent have it regularly. Fellatio is a much more common practice among gay men.[5] The idea that *all* gay men and *only* gay men have anal sex—one that the Religious Right would like us to believe—is simply not supported. Furthermore, there is no evidence that any single group defined by sexual orientation has a great deal more anal sex than any other group. In fact, depending on which survey you cite, from 20 to 45 percent of women have anal sex.[6]

Myth #6: Straight men who like anal sex are really gay.

TRUTH: Because anal sex is falsely but intrinsically linked with gay men and gay sex, there is a myth that if men want anal sex, then they must be gay. In most cases, men who identify as heterosexual and desire anal sex with women (whether they are on the giving or receiving end) are not repressing homosexual desires or tendencies. Their desire for a particular sexual activity does not rely on or "cancel out" their sexual preference in a partner. According to research, more gay men regularly practice fellatio than anal sex, and as my friend Audrey says, "How come no one ever asks: If a straight guy likes blow jobs, does that mean he's really gay?"

It's ironic: even though butt-fucking is popularly associated with gay men in today's sexual culture, it is in fact heterosexuals who have gone wild about their asses. Ask anyone who works in a sex toy shop what single item has surged forward in sales in the past fifteen years: buttplugs. And dildo harnesses for women who are clearly involved with men.

—*Susie Bright*

Myth #7: Anal sex is always painful for the person on the receiving end.

TRUTH: With desire, relaxation, communication, trust, and lots of lubrication, anal sex can be not only pain-free but arousing and orgasmic. Anal sex does not have to be painful at all, not even a little. If it is, your body is telling you that you should stop. If you ignore your body's warnings and continue, then you can hurt yourself. The experience may make you and your anus more tense the next time you try anal penetration. Your body remembers everything, so don't try to fool it.

Myth #8: Women don't enjoy receiving anal sex; they do it just to please their partners.

TRUTH: This is a particularly insidious myth about heterosexual women. Often, when we do hear about women having anal sex, the story goes something like this: The long-term boyfriend begged and begged, and finally his girlfriend gave in to his demands. Her boyfriend was pleased, but she didn't enjoy herself one bit. We never hear stories about women who crave and enjoy anal play, women who initiate anal sex, or women who are more than happy to knock on their boyfriends' back door. Sex advice columnist Susan Crain Bakos says, "Buttfucking is seen as the ultimate male sexual fantasy. We, as a culture, don't understand how much women can like taking it up the ass." [7] And, I would add, giving it up the ass as well.

Myth #9: Anal sex is the easiest way to get AIDS.

TRUTH: Because anal and rectal tissue is delicate and easily torn, viruses can be easily transmitted through the tissue into the bloodstream; so, unprotected anal intercourse with an infected person is a high-risk activity for both partners—statistically higher than vaginal intercourse with an infected person—for all STDs, including HIV.

Unprotected oral-anal contact and digital penetration also puts both partners at risk—the receiver because of fragile rectal tissue and the giver because of cuts or sores that may be on the hands or mouth. However, anal sex does not *automatically* lead to AIDS. Anal sex practiced with common sense, condoms, latex gloves, dental dams, and lube (or an HIV-negative monogamous partner) can be as safe as other sexual practices. (Read more about safer sex in chapters 2 and 4 and HIV/AIDS in chapter 11).

Myth #10: Anal sex is naughty.

TRUTH: Well, this is actually a myth *and* a truth. Of course, anal sex is not really bad for you and doesn't make you a bad person. However, for those of you who are turned on by the idea that anal sex is taboo, deviant, and naughty, don't let me ruin your party. Lots of people actually incorporate the myths I've discussed—especially the "naughtiness factor"—into their erotic anal play.

> *I love that anal sex is taboo and that not everyone admits to doing it.*

> *The taboo of anal sex gives me a rush, as well as knowing how intense it is for my partner. I love to watch her ass pounding against me.*

> *I love the idea that I am fucking my partner in the ass. It feels taboo and sexy all at the same time.*

Exercise: Personal Mythology

What did you learn about anal sex during your childhood, your teens, your adulthood? Write down everything you know about anal sex, even things you know are untrue; just let whatever comes to mind flow onto paper.

When you're finished, compare your list to the myths and truths reviewed in this chapter. Figure out what among your list is fact and what is fiction. Keep the list handy as you read the rest of the book. You may also want to repeat this exercise with a partner as part of a discussion about anal sex. By acknowledging and discussing the myths that affect our desires and fears in a safe environment, we can begin to see the truths behind the myths. One very important truth to remember is that anal sex can be safe, fun, and pleasurable.

NOTES

1. Samuel S. Janus and Cynthia L. Janus, *The Janus Report on Sexual Behavior* (New York: John Wiley & Sons, 1993), 105.

2. Jack Morin, *Anal Pleasure and Health* (San Francisco: Yes/Down There Press, 1986), 17.

3. Janus and Janus, *Janus Report;* William H. Masters, Virginia E. Johnson, and Robert E. Kolodny, *Heterosexuality* (New York: HarperCollins, 1994); Elliot Leland and Cynthia Brantley, *Sex on Campus: The Naked Truth About the Real Sex Lives of College Students* (New York: Random House, 1997); June M. Reinisch with Ruth Beasley, *The Kinsey Institute New Report on Sex* (New York: St. Martin's Press, 1990); Robert T. Michael et al., *Sex in America: A Definitive Survey* (New York: Little, Brown and Co., 1994).

4. Cathy Winks and Anne Semans, *The New Good Vibrations Guide to Sex* (San Francisco: Cleis Press, 1997), 128.

5. Morin, *Anal Pleasure,* 9 and Reinisch, Kinsey New Report, 137.

6. Leland and Brantley, *Sex on Campus;* Michael, *Sex in America;* Janus and Janus, *Janus Report;* Reinisch and Beasley, *Kinsey New Report;* Morin, *Anal Pleasure and Health.*

7. Susan Crain Bakos, *Kink: The Hidden Sex Lives of Americans* (New York: St. Martin's Press, 1995), 7.

QUOTES AND SIDEBARS

Sarah Miller, "The Slut Within," *Details* (The Sex Issue), May 1997, 77. © by Sarah Miller, reprinted with permission of the author.

Susie Bright, *Susie Bright's Sexual State of the Union* (New York: Simon & Schuster, 1997), 144.

Our Asses, Ourselves

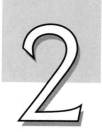

A Brief Anatomy Lesson

Although anatomy is part of science and medicine, the study of anatomy is less objective than one might think. There are a variety of differing interpretations and opinions about the internal structure of our bodies—especially the nuances and complexities of our sexual anatomy. This is certainly true for anorectal anatomy. The discussion of anatomy and the anatomical illustrations in this book are based on my interpretations of several sources, including medical textbooks, sex manuals, and conversations with sex educators.[1]

The Anus, Anal Sphincters, and PC Muscles

The anus is the external opening of the anal canal. It is comprised of folds of soft, pink tissue that give it a wrinkled or puckered appearance. The area around the

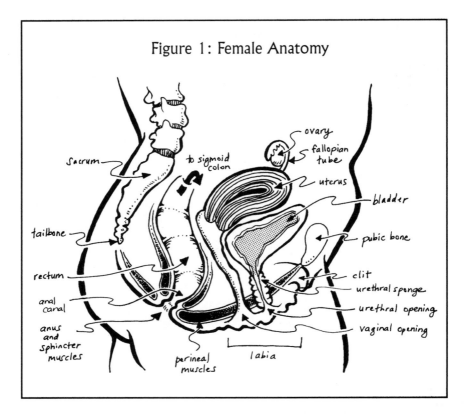

Figure 1: Female Anatomy

opening is full of hair follicles; the hair may be fine and light, coarse and dark, or somewhere in between. Everyone has hair surrounding the anus.

Rich in blood vessels and nerve endings, the tissue of the anus is incredibly sensitive and responsive to touch and stimulation. In fact, it can be one of our most sensual erogenous zones, but it is one too often feared, forgotten, and left unexplored. With regular bathing and personal hygiene, the anus is generally clean, with only trace amounts of feces, which carry bacteria from the bowels.

Two muscles—the anal sphincters—surround the anal opening (see figures 1 and 2). The external sphincter is closest to the opening. With patience and practice, you can voluntarily control the external sphincter, making it tense or relax. The internal sphincter is controlled by the autonomic nervous system, which controls involuntary bodily functions like your breathing rate. This muscle ordinarily reacts reflexively; for example, when you are ready to have a bowel movement, the internal sphincter relaxes, allowing feces to move from the rectum to the anal canal. Because the external and the internal sphincters overlap, they often work together.

Other surrounding muscles also contribute to sensations in the anal area. The perineal muscles support the area between the anus and the genitals. In this group are the pubococcygeus muscles (PC muscles), which support the pelvis from the pubic bone to the tailbone. For both men and women, these muscles contract during sexual arousal and climax; specifically, they usually contract randomly when you are aroused and rhythmically during orgasm.

I love the control I have over my ass muscles and how powerful they feel when I grip my lover's cock.

The more attention you pay to your sphincter muscles, the easier it will be to begin to relax them. Because the two muscles work in tandem, you can encourage the internal sphincter to relax by relaxing the external sphincter. Many people have found that by exercising and strengthening their PC and pelvic muscles, they can have more control of their sphincter muscles and can achieve more intense orgasms.

Exercising Your Pelvic and PC Muscles

The following exercises can help you to become more aware of your sphincter and PC muscles and learn to control and strengthen them. They will help you get in tune with the feelings in your pelvic area, increasing your sensitivity and responsiveness. The exercises will also tone the pelvic muscles, making them more flexible and more receptive to pleasurable sensations; plus, when you exercise the PC muscles, other muscles in the area also are exercised and strengthened.

You can do the exercises lying down, sitting, or standing. As with any exercise regimen, you should do them daily for best results. If your muscles seem tired at first, don't worry—that's normal. Use your common sense, and don't overdo it to begin with. The harder the exercises are to do for you, the less toned your PC muscles are, and the more you need a workout; however, if you experience any pain while doing them, see a doctor. Exercising the PC muscles during masturbation or foreplay increases blood flow in the area, thereby increasing arousal.

JAY POSITIONED HERSELF CAREFULLY over the woman's back, her arm drew back and the muscles that had lifted beams now poised for a more delicate power. She pushed her finger, blunt and strong, into Carol, feeling the tight resistance of the ass muscles, the strong sentinels protecting the soft world inside. Carol moaned, a different sound from when Jay penetrated her cunt. This was deeper, almost as if the body was finding a new voice for this more guarded entry.

—JOAN NESTLE

Women who regularly exercise their PC and pelvic muscles report some very positive benefits: heightened pelvic sensations and greater anal sensitivity; increased pleasure during clitoral stimulation, and during vaginal and anal penetration; more control over orgasms; and better, more intense orgasms. Some of the following exercises are called Kegel exercises, named for the physician who first studied PC muscles and popularized the theory of exercising them, and others are those recommended by other health care professionals.[2]

Exercise: Your PC Muscles

FINDING THEM
In order to locate your PC muscles, pretend that you are trying to stop peeing (or while you are peeing, you can actually stop the flow of urine). The muscles you contract to stop the flow are your PC muscles. If you put your finger on your perineum—the area between your vagina and your anus—while you do this exercise, you can feel the contractions.

NICE AND EASY
Take a deep breath and while you inhale, contract the muscles and hold the contraction for a few seconds. Then exhale and relax the muscles. This combination of inhale-contract and exhale-relax is what your body does naturally. For best results, you should do about a hundred repetitions per day.

QUICK AND CLEAN
Take a deep breath and this time while you inhale, tighten and release the muscles repeatedly (about ten times), then exhale and relax. Try to do these contractions as quickly as you can. Twenty to fifty sets a day is recommended.

SUCK IT IN

For this exercise, inhale and pretend you are sucking water inside your vagina and anus. Then exhale and bear down, pushing out that imaginary water. You will exercise your pelvic muscles and your stomach muscles. For best results, do ten to thirty each day.

SHAKE IT, GIRL

Renowned anal health expert Jack Morin recommends moving your body while you do your pelvic exercises:

> I suggest combining the Kegel exercises with lots of free movement in a variety of settings. The positive effects of this movement will be limited, however, if you hold your pelvis rigid while moving the rest of your body. In fact, habitual, chronic, pelvic "holding on" is one major reason why so many people need Kegel exercises. Holding the pelvis requires muscular tension which restricts movement. Restricted movement allows muscles to deteriorate.[3]

Try combining the exercises with walking, running, dancing, or simulating a hula-hoop motion.

My friend Wendy—

dirty enough to do it

but too coy to give

details—describes the

allure with vague

biology, using terms like

membrane and pressure

points. But physical

sensations are secondary.

The best part is how one

small act can make you

so dirty so fast.

—Sarah Miller

The Anal Canal and the Rectum

The anus is the opening to another responsive site of pleasure—the anal canal. The anal canal is about one to two
inches long and leads into the rectum. The same soft tissue that makes up the anus comprises the anal canal, so it
is very sensitive to touch and stimulation. The walls of the
anal canal are comprised of tissue that, like that of the
clitoris and penis, becomes engorged from increased
blood flow during arousal. When the sphincter muscles
are relaxed, these folds of tissue give the anal canal a
tremendous ability to expand. If the sphincter muscles are

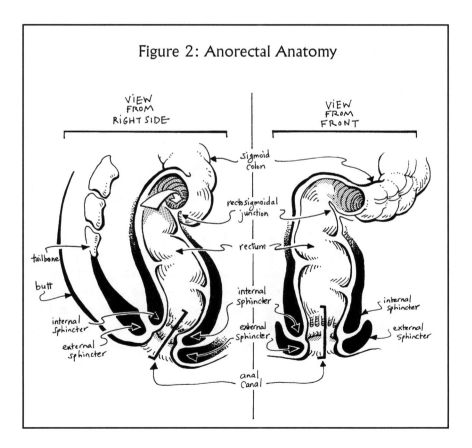

Figure 2: Anorectal Anatomy

not relaxed, and the anus is tense, penetration is possible only with force, causing tearing of the tissue and pain.

I love the feeling of surrender [when someone penetrates my ass]. The intensity. It is so much more intense than vaginal stimulation. There are so many more nerve endings in the anus. It takes me out of my head and into my body...in a way that no other type of sexual activity does. At the same time, it is not something I would do every day. Sometimes months or years go by before I am really "ready" for this type of deep stimulation.

A person's butt is as unique as a fingerprint.

—Bert Herrman

Beyond the anal canal is the rectum, which is about five inches long; the rectum is made up of loose folds of soft, smooth tissue. It, too, has a large capacity for expanding; plus it is wider than the anal canal. The rectum is tubular and curves gently (see figure 2). The lower part of the rectum curves toward your navel. After a few inches, the rectum curves back toward your spine. After another inch or so, the rectum becomes the sigmoid colon, which curves toward your navel. The rectum and colon both curve laterally (from side to side) as well; whether to the right or the left will vary from person to person. These curves are part of the reason that slowness and patience are key to pleasurable anal penetration. Each person's rectum and its curves are unique, and it is best to feel your way inside the rectum slowly, following its curves, rather than jamming anything straight inside.

Men's and women's anal anatomy is very similar, but there are some important differences (see figure 3).

The G-spot (or urethral sponge) is a raised area of tissue wrapped around the urethra in women. The urethral sponge can be found in the front wall of the vagina, and many women enjoy having it stimulated. It is most easily found and stimulated during rear-entry vaginal penetration; some women experience G-spot stimulation during anal penetration as well.

Men can experience stimulation of the prostate gland when they are anally penetrated. The prostate gland, which surrounds the urethra, is below the bladder and above the base of the penis. You can find it a few inches into the anal canal and toward the navel. This is the gland that produces semen, and it can be a big source of pleasure for men when they receive anal penetration. It is very

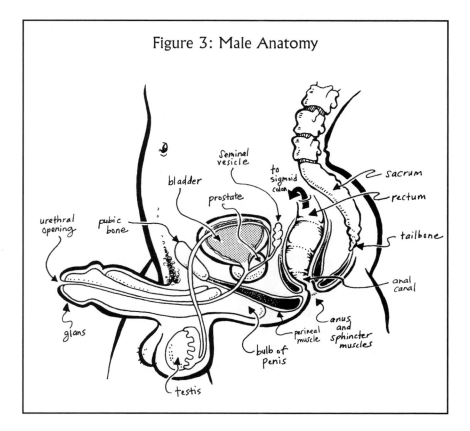

Figure 3: Male Anatomy

sensitive to massage, and most men prefer gentle rubbing; any jerky movement or poking can be very uncomfortable.

Always remember that each person's G-spot or prostate gland is unique—some people may enjoy this stimulation and others may not.

Before you experiment with anal stimulation or penetration, it is important to begin with anal exploration. In other words, you need to get more acquainted with your anus. This is not just an exercise for beginners. Most of us—even the most experienced anal sex experts—don't ever take the time to look at our own anuses.

Exercise: Take a Good Look

Get a hand-held mirror and find a suitable, well-lit place. First, take some deep breaths for several minutes to relax. Perhaps, lie down on the bed, play some soothing music, or light some incense. These are simply suggestions—do whatever things will relax *you*. Once you feel relaxed and ready to explore, find a comfortable position, one where you'll be able to stay for a while and where you'll have a good view of your butt. Begin by looking at your anus. Just check it out—the shape, the size, the color. How does it look? Relaxed, tense, somewhere in between? Gently massage your buttocks, inner thighs, and the area around your anus. Continue to massage, stroke, and explore the area, going at your own pace. Note how the opening responds to the massage around it. When you feel comfortable, gently touch your anus. Don't penetrate it, just do some external touching. Tune into the sensations you feel, both in your anus and in the rest of your body. Keep touching, but just touching—no penetration of any kind yet—and when you feel like stopping, stop. Some people may like to write down some thoughts in a journal about the experience to refer to later.

Basic Preparations

The following are some basic preparations for having safe and pleasurable anal sex. (I will discuss more about safer sex as it pertains to STDs and HIV/AIDS in chapters 4 and 11.)

Short, Smooth Nails

The tissue of the anus, anal canal, and rectum is very delicate, much more delicate than the tissue of the vagina. In order to make stimulation and penetration comfortable for yourself and your partner, make sure your nails are short and filed smooth, with no jagged or sharp edges. Even if you plan to wear latex gloves—and you should—it's a good idea to make sure those nails don't become daggers cloaked in latex inside your partner's ass (or your own!). Short, smooth nails will help prevent small tears in the anal tissue, which can cause irritation and discomfort during anal play and bowel movements.

Clean Tools

Anything you plan to put in an anus should be cleaned beforehand. Your hands, and, if applicable, your partner's hands or penis should be thoroughly washed in hot water and a good antibacterial soap. Toys like butt plugs and dildos should also be cleaned with hot water and soap; in addition, you should soak toys for about fifteen minutes to disinfect them with either povidone iodine (Betadine), hydrogen peroxide (full strength), bleach (diluted: one part bleach, ten parts water), or a sex toy cleaner you can purchase where sex toys are sold. Alternatively (or in addition), you can put a new condom on each toy (including your partner's penis) before using it and a new latex glove on your hand, which can be discarded after each use. Using latex not only ensures that everything is safe and clean for sex play but also makes for easier cleanup during and after sex. (For more about latex and condoms, see the "Latex" section in chapter 4.)

One very important thing to remember is that once anything—a finger, a toy, a penis—has been in the anus, it must be thoroughly washed or covered with a new condom or latex glove before it goes anywhere near the vagina. Putting something in an ass and then transferring it directly to the vagina is a perfect route to vaginal infections, including yeast infections, urinary tract infections, and other bacterial baddies. So, please, just don't go there before getting clean! In addition, sex researchers Masters and Johnson report that washing the penis may not be enough to prevent gastrointestinal bacteria from the rectum from transferring to the vagina because "there may be bacteria scooped inside the urethra which escape the cleansing action of soap and water."[4] Another smart reason to use a new condom for each new journey—and for both women and men to urinate after any penetrative sex.

Clean Butt and Empty Bowels

The best way to have a happy and healthy rectum is to make sure you eat enough fiber; if, however, your butt is feeling under the weather, it's a good idea to postpone anal erotic activity until things are back to normal. It's ideal to have a bowel movement before you plan to have anal sex of any kind, because empty bowels tend to make anal erotic experiences more comfortable for everyone. Feces are stored in the colon. They pass into the rectum when the body prepares for a bowel movement. If you have a bowel movement shortly after you feel the urge, feces pass through the rectum and anal canal and out of your body. (Many people cannot or do not go to the bathroom at that moment and instead "hold it in." In this case, feces then remain in the rectum.) After a bowel movement, there is normally only a trace amount of fecal matter in the anal canal and rectum; however, if you have a poor diet, recurring constipation, diarrhea, or other intestinal disorders, there may be more fecal matter present than usual. In any case, remember that even the healthiest rectum contains some fecal matter, which carries bacteria from the colon—E. coli bacteria, as well as hepatitis A, parasites, amoebas, or viruses that may be present.

Some people like to take a shower or bath before sex to clean the anal area. I know a warm, soapy shower reassures me that my ass is clean for my partner's tongue, fingers, penis, or toys and makes me less self-conscious about having anal sex. You may also want to have an enema, although enemas are not necessary for having safe, fun, and relatively clean anal sex. (Read more about enemas in chapter 5.)

Relaxation

It is so important for both partners to be relaxed in order to have healthy, sensuous anal sex. Remember that you can relax all the muscle groups in the anal area, and when they're not relaxed, anal sex—in fact, any anal activity, including a bowel movement—can be uncomfortable, if not downright painful. Fear, stress, and tension can all be felt intensely in your ass. When your mind and body are relaxed, focused on pleasure, and ready to experience anal eroticism, the encounter will be that much more satisfying. I recommend a lot of touching, caressing, massaging, kissing, and sweet-talking leading up to anal sex. Get rid of all external distractions and set the stage: shut off the ringer on the phone, put on some sexy music, light some candles, make the bed with special sheets, wear something sexy. Do whatever it takes to put you and your partner in the mood. Then take your time. I find that extensive touching of the entire body, touching that's not necessarily sexual or genitally focused, is a great way to relax both body and mind and really prepares you to hone in on all your senses. A warm bubble bath is also a good way to relax the body, get in the mood, and get your bottom nice and clean for that special someone.

Safety First

Let me define some of the terms I will use throughout this book in discussing safer sex:

You may be *monogamous* with your partner. You have committed to be each other's sole sexual partner. You've been tested for HIV and STDs, and you do not necessarily use latex barriers or follow safer sex guidelines.

Or, you may be in a *fluid-bonded, nonmonogamous* relationship. You have committed to practice safer sex with any sexual contacts other than your partner. You've been tested for HIV and STDs. When you have sex with each other, you do not normally use latex barriers or condoms, and you do come into contact with each other's bodily fluids. When you have sex with others, you always practice safer sex.

You may be *nonmonogamous*. You may have multiple partners with whom you may (or may not) enter into relationships. Regardless of whether you have one partner or many, if you have not been tested recently for all STDs, do not know your partners' sexual histories and practices *and* your partners' partners' sexual histories and practices, do not know your HIV status, or do not know your partners' HIV status, you should follow safer sex guidelines designed to prevent transmission of HIV and other diseases.

Naturally, if you have an STD or HIV, you will want to follow safer sex guidelines at all times.

Unless you are monogamous or fluid-bonded, your sexual repertoire should involve safer sex practices to prevent sexually transmitted diseases and HIV/AIDS—anal sex is no exception to this rule. In fact, because of the delicacy of anal and rectal tissue, bodily fluids infected with HIV and other viruses are transmitted and absorbed easily and quickly into the bloodstream through the mucous membrane of the rectum. Thus, unprotected anal intercourse can be more risky for both partners than unprotected vaginal intercourse.

For those of you in monogamous or fluid-bonded relationships, The American Medical Women's Association recommends that before safer sex precautions are discontinued, both you and your partner be tested for HIV three to six months after either of you has had sexual contact with another partner.[5] If you and your partner are monogamous or fluid-bonded and have both tested negative for all STDs and HIV, you can still utilize safer sex practices for anal sex. As you'll read in chapter 4, latex barriers and lubricants help prevent not only the spread of STDs and HIV but also the spread of bacteria from the bowels. In general, latex and lubricants make anal play easier in lots of different ways.

If you are nonmonogamous or do not know your HIV or STD status (or your partner's) you should practice safer sex, using condoms and latex gloves for anal sex—and for all sexual activities in which you may come into contact with your partner's bodily fluids—to prevent the transmission of STDs and HIV.

Nonoxynol-9, which is found in some lubricants and some lubricated condoms, is a chemical proven to kill HIV (the virus that causes AIDS) and other STD viruses in laboratory tests. Although it is widely recommended that nonoxynol-9 be used during vaginal intercourse, many women find that they are allergic to nonoxynol-9; it irritates their vaginas and causes vaginal infections. There are differing opinions about its use for anal intercourse.

There is not enough research on the effects of nonoxynol-9 on rectal tissue or for anal sex, and my research illustrates the multiple opinions about it. *The Women's HIV Source Book* and *The American Medical Women's Association Guide to Sexuality* recommend that you always use nonoxynol-9 for intercourse; however, neither book indicates any specifics for vaginal versus anal penetration.[6] *The Kinsey Institute New Report on Sex* does advocate the use of nonoxynol-9 in anal intercourse and has no discussion of possible risks or side effects.[7]

The New Good Vibrations Guide to Sex as well as a supervisor I interviewed at San Francisco Sex Information both recommend that you *not* use nonoxynol-9 for anal intercourse because of the delicacy of the rectal tissue. These sources agree with the many people who believe that nonoxynol-9 may be too harsh and irritating for the delicate tissue of the anal canal and rectum. Because it's likely to irritate or traumatize the rectal tissue, it may actually make transmission of HIV faster and easier, providing the virus with an accessible route to the bloodstream.[8]

If you are using your fingers or a sex toy for penetration and make sure to use a new glove or condom each time, using a lubricant without nonoxynol-9 is pretty safe. If, however, your partner is a man and you want him to penetrate you with his penis, I recommend using a condom and plenty of lube and having your partner withdraw before ejaculation. That way, if the condom breaks or leaks and you don't have nonoxynol-9 as a backup, semen (which could be infected) will be outside your body instead of inside your delicate rectum.[9] *The Complete Guide to Safer Sex* from the Institute for Advanced Study of Human Sexuality offers another tip:

> Nonoxynol-9 lubricated condoms have only been tested for vaginal intercourse. Accordingly, some using them for anal intercourse may wish to put the condom on then wipe off the outside so as to have added protection on the inside of the condom without using it on anal tissue.[10]

Unless you are monogamous or fluid-bonded, your male partner should always wear a condom for penis-anus penetration. (Read more about latex, lube, and safer sex in chapter 4).

A note about having anal sex while you are pregnant. Dr. Ruth Westheimer points out that some men think that having vaginal intercourse during pregnancy will somehow hurt the baby, so they suggest anal intercourse.[11] It is safe to have anal sex if you are pregnant, although some women find that they cannot get in a comfortable position for anal stimulation. Pregnant women should also be extra careful to prevent the spread of bacteria from the anus and rectum to the vagina, since vaginal infections during pregnancy can be both harder to treat and more serious.

NOTES

1. Jack Morin, *Anal Pleasure and Health* (San Francisco: Yes Press, 1986); Cathy Winks and Anne Semans, *The New Good Vibrations Guide to Sex* (San Francisco: Cleis Press, 1997); Roselyn Payne Epps and Susan Cobb Stewart, eds., *The American Medical Women's Association Guide to Sexuality* (New York: Dell Books, 1996); James H. Grendell, M.D., Kenneth R. McQuaid, M.D., and Scott L. Friedman, M.D., eds., *Current Diagnosis and Treatment in Gastroenterology* (New York: Simon & Schuster, 1996); and San Francisco sex educator Robert Morgan, personal conversations.

2. These exercises are recommended in *Anal Pleasure and Health* by Jack Morin and *The Complete Guide to Safer Sex* from the Institute for Advanced Study of Human Sexuality, edited by Ted McIlvenna (Fort Lee, NJ: Barricade Books, 1992).

3. Morin, *Anal Pleasure,* 59.

4. Masters et al., *Heterosexuality,* 384.

5. Roselyn Payne Epps and Susan Cobb Stewart, eds., *The American Medical Women's Association Guide to Sexuality* (New York: Dell Books, 1996), 158.

6. Patricia Kloser and Jane MacLean Craig, *The Women's HIV Sourcebook* (Dallas, TX: Taylor Publishing Co., 1994), 75; Epps and Stewart, *Guide to Sexuality,* 158.

7. Reinisch and Beasley, *Kinsey New Report,* 591.

8. Phone interview with San Francisco Sex Information Supervisor, May 1997; and Winks and Semans, *New Good Vibrations Guide,* 73.

9. Paul Harding Douglas and Laura Pinsky, *The Essential AIDS Fact Book* (New York: Pocket Books, 1996), 28.

10. McIlvenna, *Complete Guide to Safer Sex,* 84. This tip assumes that the condom is lubricated on both the inside and the outside.

11. Dr. Ruth Westheimer, *Sex for Dummies*™ (Braintree, MA: IDG Books Worldwide, 1995), 182.

QUOTES AND SIDEBARS

Joan Nestle, "A Different Place" in *A Restricted Country* (Ithaca, NY: Firebrand Books, 1987), 137. ©1987 by Joan Nestle. Reprinted with permission of the author and Firebrand Books.

Sarah Miller, "The Slut Within," *Details (The Sex Issue),* May 1997, 77. ©1997 by Sarah Miller. Reprinted with permission of the author.

Bert Herrman, *Trust: The Hand Book (A Guide to the Sensual and Spiritual Art of Handballing)* (San Francisco: Alamo Square Press, 1991), 45.

Beyond Our Bodies:

Emotional and Psychological Aspects of Anal Eroticism

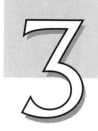

In addition to taking care of our bodies in preparation for and during anal sex, we also have to take care of other aspects of ourselves. Our emotional, psychological, and spiritual well-being play a major role in our erotic experiences, and our experiences of anal sexuality are no exception.

Desire

> The most important thing, the single most important thing when you're talking about wanting to progress forward with any kind of anal erotic play is desire. You must, must do this because you want to do it.[1]

In her positive and sexy video about anal eroticism, sex educator/porn star Nina Hartley makes this important point from the beginning: you've got to want it. There really is no faking it in anal sex. Your body, mind, and psyche all must be in agreement that you want to have anal sex. Don't have anal sex because you think it's what your partner wants. Or because your partner is pressuring you to do it. Or because you're afraid that you won't be a desirable lover if you don't do it. Take responsibility for your erotic likes and dislikes—figure out what they are and then communicate them to your partner.

No lover is able to look into your eyes and figure out how you want to get fucked in the ass.

—Susie Bright

Communication

I really like receiving, and wish I could assure my partner that if we're doing it right, it won't hurt, and that it'll feel good. Also, my current partner is very worried about fecal matter, so I wish I had some way of addressing that.

Communication is a key component before, during, and after anal sex. It's a good idea to talk to your partner about anal eroticism, sharing your desires and fantasies as well as your fears, *before* you go knocking on that back door. In fact, I think it's best if you discuss it with your partner in a nonsexual setting, rather than *right* before you're about to delve into anal erotic play. When bringing up the subject, you might test the waters in a playful, positive way; see what your partner thinks about the subject in general, then about you doing it in particular.

The hotel had been closed for months and we broke in to fuck. He was a big guy, hairy, not my type at all. But the way he handled me was magnificent. And he asked permission to fuck my ass. Good sexual manners go a long way with me.

Fear

> The ass is a gift. When a woman kneels with her ass in the air, head well down, she feels erotic dread grow in the pit of her stomach and spread through her loins. She can want for this and fear it. In my anticipation of the entry thrust, my heart beats faster, the walls of my vagina swell. It's all up to him. How will he take me?[2]

People have a lot of fears and negative feelings about anal eroticism. Some of these feelings stem from our society's myths and taboos about anal sex. Myths about anal sex being unnatural, perverted, dirty, painful, and dangerous have become very real fears in people's minds. It is important to realize that we are all made aware of the anal taboo and myths starting in childhood and therefore we are all affected in some way by them.

AS THE RECEPTIVE PARTNER, WHAT ARE YOUR FEARS?
> *My lover will think I'm weird for wanting to do it.*
> *It will be too tight for his penis to fit.*
> *I'll get hemorrhoids.*
> *It will be messy, and my butt will smell bad.*
> *I'll get constipated or have diarrhea.*
> *It will hurt, something will get ruptured.*
> *It won't feel good—I won't like it.*
> *I won't be able to take her dildo.*
> *I'll get an STD or another disease.*

AS THE INSERTIVE PARTNER, WHAT ARE YOUR FEARS?
> *I'll hurt my partner or make her bleed.*
> *It will be dirty, and I'll get shit on me.*
> *I won't do it right.*
> *I won't like it.*

My lover will think I'm weird for wanting to do it.
I'll get an STD or another disease.
My boyfriend is worried that people will think he's gay.

While most of these fears have their roots in myths and misconceptions about anal sex, it is important to respect and validate your partner when she or he shares her or his fears. Talk with your partner about fears you both have, and review the chapter on myths, dispelling the misinformation and replacing it with correct information. Reassure each other that either one of you can stop activity at any time and be fully supported by the other one. Set concrete ground rules and boundaries about what is okay and what isn't; as experiences progress, the boundaries can change if needed. Each person needs to know that she or he will be safe from both pain and disease during anal sex and that there is mutual trust and respect.

Fear and tension that are not articulated and resolved will ultimately be felt in your anus, which will be tense and unwilling. Nina Hartley reminds us, "Of all the parts of your body, nothing knows a liar like your anus. So if your mind is saying 'Yes! Yes!' and your heart is saying 'No! No!' your anus will always listen to your heart."[3]

Expectations, Needs, and Fantasies

Having an open, honest discussion can help illuminate what each person wants from the experience and why, so both people are less likely to make incorrect assumptions about the other person's desires and expectations. You can ask each other, What do you want? What do you expect? What are your needs?

It will feel okay, but I'll never want to do it again.
I want to work my way up to one finger, then stop.

Let's try just external stimulation, nothing inside.
I'd like licking and touching, but no penetration.
I want to be able to have the small dildo in my butt.
We've done fingers a dozen times, tonight I want your cock.
I want everything to feel safe.

What have your previous experiences been with anal eroticism? Share them, discuss them. Why do you want to explore anal sensuality?

I want to explore something new with my partner.
I'm curious about what it feels like.
I've done it before and want to do it again.
You want to do it and I don't want to say no to you.
I want to feel closer to my lover.
It's something special and intimate and something I want to share with my partner.
I saw it in a porn movie, it turned me on, and I want to try it.
It's always been a fantasy of mine.

Fantasies can be incredibly powerful forces in our lives, erotic and otherwise. Many people fantasize about erotic activities like anal sex but are afraid to vocalize their desires. The myths and misinformation about anal sex contribute to the silence and sometimes prevent us from satisfying our curiosities. Sharing our sexual fantasies with a partner can deepen a sexual relationship and help us communicate our needs and desires.

It is equally important to distinguish our fantasies from our realities. If your favorite masturbatory fantasy involves someone ramming your butt repeatedly with a swollen silicone dick that makes you come every time, don't be surprised if you don't get the same result when you try it out. There are some fantasies that we can share and help bring to life and others that should probably remain fantasies. Have realistic expectations for yourself and know the limits of your own body, especially when it comes to anal sex. One finger in your anus and a whisper in your ear about that big dick might just do the trick.

During the experience, talk to each other, find out what feels good and what doesn't, what's working and what's not.

How does this feel?

Would you like more or less movement?

Do you want me to play with your pussy while I'm doing your ass?

How is this position?

That feels great—keep doing it.

I love doing this to you.

Do you want another finger now?

I want you to lick my ass.

Afterward, have a little debriefing session to review how it went and get feedback you can use for next time. Remind each other about goals you set. Did I go too fast, did I use enough lube? Was there enough in-and-out movement, or do you want more of just that pressure feeling? What did you like about my fingers versus the butt plug? Is there something I can do differently next time? Do you want more genital stimulation while I'm playing with your butt? Compliments always feel good—criticism does not. Be generous when you communicate with your partner. If you want to tell her or him about something you didn't like, why not start that conversation with something you did like? But make sure you do talk about what wasn't pleasurable as well as what was pleasurable. Communication at all phases of an anal sex experience will ultimately help both partners to articulate their needs, and, ideally, help everyone get what they want out of anal sex.

Patience

Patience is crucial. Everyone must go at their own pace for anal sex to be pleasurable. When both partners are patient, it's much easier for both, especially the receptive partner, to relax. Anal sex is also a gradual process of exploration. Unlike in those hot anal sex porn videos some of us love to watch, you really can't jump right from kissing to having a hard cock—flesh or silicone—in your ass. Remember, those are professional actors in the videos. Keep in mind that they have had extensive experience with anal penetration, and they, too, start with a few fingers or a small butt plug before that dick just slides right in. Even in amateur videos, as well as in the more professional ones, the actors' preparation is happening off camera or ends up on the editor's cutting room floor. In real life and real time, we *progress* to anal penetration. Anal sex is not a choice activity for a night when you just want a quickie, or someone has somewhere to be. If you are nervous, anxious, or stressed out about anal sex, sex in general, or the presentation you're giving tomorrow at work, it's probably not the best time to experience anal eroticism.

Presence

Speaking of communication and patience, it's best to be sober if you're going to engage in anal play—although I'm not going to preach about it or deny that people combine alcohol and drugs and pleasurable anal sex.

Many people find that drugs, especially volatile nitrites ("poppers") help them relax during anal intercourse. Inhaling volatile nitrites, such as amyl-nitrite and isobutyl, causes your blood vessels to dilate and your blood pressure to drop and gives you a "rush" feeling as your body tries to stabilize itself.

I believe that with proper relaxation, communication, trust, and desire, people can experience pleasurable anal intercourse without drugs; ultimately, alcohol and drugs of any kind alter your awareness of your body, an awareness you absolutely must have to enjoy anal sex. People are more likely to ignore their anal boundaries—both physical and mental—if their judgment is impaired by alcohol and drugs. Anal sex requires both partners to have patience, skill, good communication, and coordination. The insertive partner needs to be keenly aware, intuitive, and able to read her or his partner's body lan-

THEIR PENISES MOVED IN UNISON INSIDE ME. I could clearly feel them both, their tips meeting, brushing each other through what felt like a flimsy membrane, a thin wall of skin which was in danger at every thrust, and was becoming more and more fragile. They're going to tear me, I thought, they're going to tear me and then they really will meet, one against the other. I repeated it to myself. I liked hearing myself say it. They're going to tear me. What a delicious idea...

—ALMUDENA GRANDES

guage and nonverbal cues. The receiver needs to be in touch with his or her body to know what feels good and what doesn't. I believe that all this is more easily achieved when both people are sober.

Trust and Power

> I like the sense that I'm breaking and entering, overtaking and existing inside someone else's body.

A sexual interaction like anal sex, in which one person gives their body over to another, can raise deep issues of power and trust. The power dynamics can be especially magnified during anal sex because it is such a forbidden act and because of the physical delicacy of the anus and rectum. Anal sex can be very charged, intense, and emotional:

> I like the full-up feeling, sometimes, which I get both from being fucked and being fingered while my vagina is also being entered and my clit is being played with. Sometimes I want intercourse to…feel overwhelming, and anal intercourse feels like this. I associate receiving anal sex with submission, but also with toughness, being able to take it.

It's important for partners to be able to discuss their feelings openly, feel safe, and trust one another. The person receiving anal penetration can feel especially vulnerable, both physically and emotionally, and the partner giving anal pleasure must respect the receiver's wishes, needs, and limits. The giver may fear that she or he will hurt the receiving partner and needs to be reassured that everyone is dedicated to making it not hurt.

Again, communication and ground rules can help alleviate tension and reassure both people that it will be a pain-free, safe experience.

> I love feeling arms and legs around me, totally enveloped, while someone I love and trust is in my ass and playing with my clit and licking my ear. It's like feeling safe and loved but vulnerable and sexy all at the same time. I can't imagine doing it with someone I didn't trust deeply and feel strongly about. It seems more intimate than vaginal sex.

The intimacy, intensity, and ecstasy of anal pleasure can sometimes be overwhelming, but it can also be very special and extremely satisfying.

> The person I've "given" to had never given or received ever before herself...It was new and exciting for her, and it showed that she trusted me and cared about me enough to try it...She knew it was something I enjoyed, and she let me share it with her.

NOTES
1. Nina Hartley, *Nina Hartley's Guide to Anal Sex* (Adam and Eve Productions, 1994). This video is available at many adult video and sex toy stores and through mail-order catalogs. See the resource section at the end of the book for more information.
2. Bakos, *Kink,* 10.
3. Hartley, *Guide to Anal Sex.*

QUOTES AND SIDEBARS
Susie Bright, "Ass Forward" in *Susie Sexpert's Lesbian Sex World* (San Francisco: Cleis Press, 1990), 34. ©1990 by Susie Bright.
Almudena Grandes, *The Ages of Lulu,* translated by Sinia Soto (New York: Grove Press, 1994), 184.

Tools of the Trade

4

There are plenty of toys and other tools you can use to enhance anal pleasure. Many products are designed and marketed especially for anal sex, and others used for vaginal stimulation and penetration can also be used anally (see figure 4). When choosing a toy, you should decide on what sensation you'd like to experience: Do you want something in your ass for a "full" feeling? Do you want in-out fucking similar to vaginal intercourse? Do you want what's in your ass to move or vibrate? As a general rule, all the toys discussed in this chapter should be used with lubricant and latex, which is why these are the two tools covered first. In addition to patience, relaxation, and trust, latex and lube are the most important ingredients for making anal play safe and pleasurable.

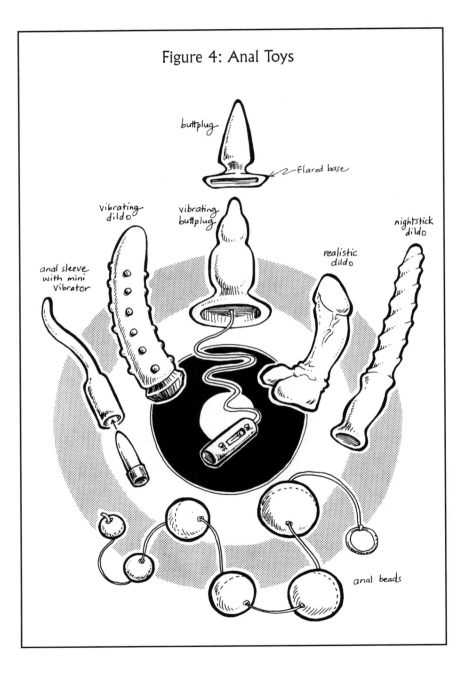

Figure 4: Anal Toys

Latex

Whether it's a tongue, a finger, a penis, or a dildo, slipping it into its own little latex outfit is always a good idea prior to an anal journey; latex makes anal sex both safer and more pleasurable. Even though too many popular safer sex guidelines for women focus only on vaginal contact, the standards for safer vaginal sex also apply to safer anal sex. If you're going to have oral-anal contact, a square piece of latex called a dental dam or a condom cut lengthwise provides a safe barrier between partners. A tip to make rimming with latex more pleasurable: use a dab of lubricant on the side facing the anus for added sensitivity.

Remember that anal and rectal tissue is very delicate and much easier to irritate and abrade than the tissue of the vaginal walls. For finger-anus penetration, the penetrator should wear either a finger cot or a latex glove and use plenty of lubricant; a stray jagged nail not properly trimmed and filed can do more damage in an anus than you might think.

As in vaginal intercourse, condoms are key to preventing the transmission of STDs and HIV during anal intercourse. Although anal

Some people like to wear butt plugs under their clothing throughout the day. We've certainly sold our share of plugs to customers who immediately take their new purchase off to the bathroom to pop it in place. Keep this possibility in mind next time an intimidating highway patrolman pulls you over—perhaps he's sitting on something that throbs even harder than his motorcycle.

—*Cathy Winks and Anne Semans*

sex involving a penis won't lead to pregnancy, it is much easier to transmit a sexually transmitted disease, especially HIV, during penis-anus intercourse, because tears in rectal tissue give semen (and whatever the semen may be carrying) direct access to the bloodstream.

Recently, a condom for women called the Reality™ Female Condom has become available (see figure 5). Marketed primarily for vaginal intercourse, the female condom is a tube of polyurethane closed at one end and open at the other, like a larger version of the male condom. Although some women find them cumbersome, others say it gives them a sense of control and responsibility in the practice of safer sex.

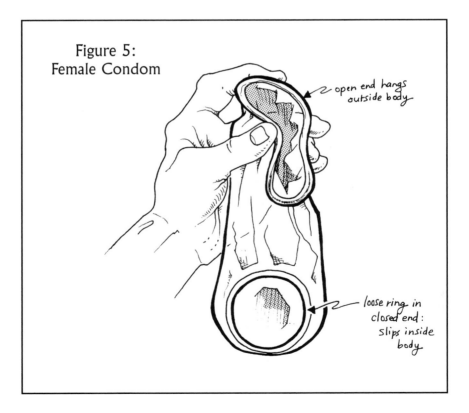

Figure 5:
Female Condom

open end hangs outside body

loose ring in closed end: slips inside body

The female condom can also be used for anal intercourse, and, in fact, it offers more protection because it
lines the anal cavity, covering the penis and the outer area
of the anus. Some people also use the female condom for
anal-oral contact, although its effectiveness for analingus
has not been scientifically tested or proven. You should
not use it for anal fisting. The female condom can be
slipped into the anus any time before penetration.

Before insertion, lubricate the outside of the condom,
and make sure that the lubrication is evenly spread by rubbing the sides of the pouch together. To insert it, squeeze
the sheath, and, starting with the inner ring, slip it into the
anus. Make sure that the inner ring is at the closed end of
the pouch. Once it is inside, push it the rest of the way with
your finger past the sphincter muscles. About an inch of the
condom should hang outside the anus, so the outer ring
doesn't slip inside during the action.

During penetration, the condom may move around,
either side to side or up and down. This is normal.
However, if your partner's penis or dildo is long or thrusts
deeply, the condom could slip all the way into the anus.
If your partner withdraws completely in between thrusts,
she or he could slip back inside your anus—but outside
the protection of the condom. If it does, stop and adjust
it. Like everything else, using the female condom takes
practice and patience. To take the condom out, squeeze
and twist the outer ring (to keep fluid inside the pouch)
and pull it out slowly and gently. Don't flush the Reality™
Female Condom in the toilet—throw it away.[1]

Latex in combination with a lubricant makes penetration smoother and easier for both partners, especially
for the person on the receiving end of penetration; of
course, the smoother things go, the more pleasurable the
experience is for both partners. And, for the person on
the giving end who may be squeamish about running into

some fecal matter while inside her or his partner's rectum, dental dams and condoms provide a good barrier.

Putting a latex glove on your hand and a condom on whatever tools you play with also keeps your hand and tools clean. You should never, ever put anything in the vagina that has been in the anus without thoroughly washing and disinfecting it first. Transferring rectal bacteria into the vagina can lead to yeast infections, urinary tract infections, and other ailments that will put a halt to your sex life. Just don't go there. If you're likely to want to use the same hand or tool in both the vagina and the anus, or your anus and then your partner's, you can avoid a lot of running to the bathroom to wash up each time you want to switch gears by using a new glove or condom each time you switch orifices or activities. Some people like to practice "double-gloving," wearing two gloves; when they are finished with one orifice, they can simply

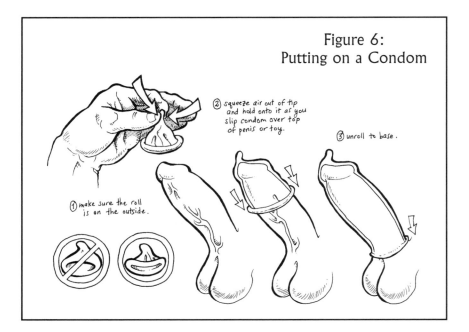

Figure 6:
Putting on a Condom

② squeeze air out of tip and hold onto it as you slip condom over top of penis or toy.

③ unroll to base.

① make sure the roll is on the outside.

peel off the top glove to reveal a fresh one underneath for the next orifice with no break in the action.

A few tips on using condoms correctly (also see figure 6):

- Latex condoms are safer, more effective barriers than animal skin or "natural" condoms.
- Don't use condoms that are ribbed or textured for anal sex; they may cause irritation or abrasions to the rectal tissue.
- Store condoms in a cool, dry place away from sunlight.
- If you use a condom with a receptacle tip, gently press the air out of the closed end before putting it on. Air bubbles rupture condoms. If you use a condom with a plain end, leave about an inch of air-free space at the tip of the condom; semen needs somewhere to go and ejaculation without that space can cause a condom to break.
- Putting a small amount of lube on the inside tip of the condom will reduce air bubbles and increase sensitivity. (Lube with nonoxynol-9 on the inside of a condom will also give you an extra measure of safety.)
- Don't reuse condoms.
- Hold onto the base of the condom when necessary, and especially during withdrawal, so it doesn't slip off.[2]
- Make sure condoms aren't old—check the expiration date.

Lubricants

Before I slide down this particular pole, let me reveal a bias: I am a firm believer that lube makes *any* sexual activity much more pleasurable. The wetter and slipperier everything is, the better. But lubricant is not just desirable; it's essential to any anal penetration. Unlike the vagina, the anus and rectum are not self-lubricating.

During anal exploration of yourself or a partner, you might find that the anus feels wet. What you're feeling is a natural mucous secretion from the anal canal and maybe some sweat—but neither this nor spit provides enough wetness to do the trick. Beyond sneaking a finger a millimeter inside someone's ass, YOU NEED LUBE.

Besides, you're already using latex and don't want it to break or tear. Nonlubricated penetration causes friction and is likely to wreak havoc on both latex and the thin, delicate anal tissue. Lube makes entry smoother and easier for both partners reducing the chance of tearing, discomfort, or pain. When the person being penetrated is comfortable, she or he can relax more easily and usually have longer, more pleasurable anal sessions.

There are many different varieties of lubricants on the market, with the widest selections at adult bookstores, sex toy shops, and mail-order catalogs. You can also check out the major drug stores. The best thing to do is to buy some sample sizes of a few different brands and experiment with them to see what's right for you and your partner. Here's a description of some of the different types of lubes:

WATER-BASED "LIQUIDY" LUBES
These slick, wet lubes are nonirritating, nonstaining, odorless, and tasteless; they are very popular for vaginal sex because they have a very similar consistency to natural vaginal secretions and are easy to wash off toys and bodies. These lubes are thin and liquidy, and a little amount tends to go a long way. Some people complain that water-based lubes dry up fast, but you can simply add a little water or saliva to revive their powers. Most of these lubes can be found in sex toy stores and catalogs, and a few, like AstroGlide and K-Y's new liquid lube, often pop up at the chain drug stores. Examples: AstroGlide,

Wet Light, Aqua Lube, Slippery Stuff, Probe Silky Light, Eros Bodyglide, K-Y Liquid.

WATER-BASED THICKER LUBES
These lubes have the same properties and advantages as their thinner counterparts. The only difference is in their consistency; they tend to feel more like hair gel or jelly. Many people like to use these thicker lubes for anal play because they provide extensive lubrication and tend to dry up less quickly than watery varieties. Examples: K-Y Jelly, Probe, ForPlay, Embrace, Elbow Grease, Wet, I-D.

OIL-BASED LUBES
Crisco isn't just for baking cookies. Crisco is a longtime favorite lubricant of gay and bisexual men (and some women) who practice anal fisting. It's inexpensive, readily available at your local supermarket, and, since it's vegetable shortening, it naturally flushes out of the rectum. Oil-based lubes don't evaporate and dry up the way water-based lubes do. The most important thing to know about oil-based lubes is that they break down latex and can eventually create very small holes in your latex condoms, gloves, and dental dams, rendering them ineffective as barriers. Never use oil-based lubes with condoms worn by a male partner; if you use an oil-based lube with a condom over a toy, you still need to clean and disinfect the toy before and after play, because pinprick holes can allow body fluids to pass through the latex onto the toy. Latex gloves are usually thicker than condoms and break down less quickly in the presence of oil-based lubes; I recommend that if you use oil-based lubes with gloves, you change into a fresh glove every fifteen to twenty minutes. Even better, reserve their use for anal play by yourself or with a monogamous or fluid-bonded partner. Oil-based lubricants are harder to wash out of the body, and they should never be used in or

*A*GAIN AND AGAIN YOUR PALM COMES DOWN ON ME, *warming, reddening my ass. Then I feel the meaner cut of a leather strap, causing me to yell and jerk with each blow. I lie tensely, expecting the next blow, and am surprised by the cold, lubed wetness of your latex-covered hand, prodding between my ass cheeks.*

"Come on boy. Open up now. Open up for me. This is where daddies get to go."

Your soothing words allow my muscles to go slack and you slide a finger slowly into my ass. It hurts at first but as you gently maneuver inside me, rubbing and lightly prodding, I find myself moving into your hand, helping you to go in further. But then you pull out, making me whimper, making me almost cry with disappointment.

"Shh, shh...you've been so good that Daddy has a little present for you."

I feel you push the smooth rubber of a medium-sized ass plug into me and I moan with the sensation.

"Now can you hold that in for a while?"

Bleary I whisper, "I think so Daddy."

— *DORIAN KEY*

around the vagina. They provide an opportune environment for bacteria and viruses to grow and thrive there.[3] Examples: Crisco, Vaseline, baby oil.

Butt Plugs

Made of silicone, latex, or vinyl, butt plugs come in many different sizes, but they all have a similar shape with slight variations: they are usually narrowest at the top, thickest in the middle, and narrow at the base, which is flared. Some are diamond shaped, others are rippled with segments going from small to large. The great thing about butt plugs is that they were made for your butt. The flared base ensures that a plug won't get "lost" or go too far inside the rectum.

Butt plugs can be inserted in the anus and worn for a period of time. Because of their shape, they are designed to stay in place rather than be pushed in and out as the sphincter muscles close around the narrow bottom. They give your ass a feeling of fullness. Butt plugs provide a great way to get your ass used to having something in it; the longer the plug stays in, the more the anal muscles tend to relax and open up. Using a series of different sizes of plugs can help you work up to having something larger in your anus, like a dildo or penis. Some people like to have a plug inside their anus while their partner stimulates their genitals or other areas of the body. There are harnesses on the market that help keep plugs in place so you can actually "wear" one for an extended amount of time. If your partner loves having her nipples sucked while her ass is fucked, or if you want to concentrate on sucking his penis and he wants something up his butt, you could feel like you're playing Twister. A butt plug is a great solution!

You may purchase the smallest plug available in order to be realistic and then find it's too small. I've heard plenty of stories from women who insert a slim plug only to have it slip out—or even shoot out across the room—at a crucial moment. If this happens to you, you don't necessarily have to run back to the store for a bigger one. If you've been doing your pelvic muscle exercises, your sphincter muscles should be strong enough to hold the plug in. (In fact, your partner "making" you hold a plug inside your ass can be a fun and sexy exercise itself.) Many of us can contract our muscles around the plug and grip it. Others may want to start with a slimmer size to warm up, then find a medium-sized one for extended plug play.

Vibrators

I just got a really nice expandable vibrating butt plug. It's a little on the large size and will take some getting used to, but the vibrations are quite powerful and its potential for use is incredible.

For people who like stimulation of those fabulous nerve endings in the anal area, vibrators can really do the trick. There are vibrators made especially for external stimulation of the genital area that work for stimulation of the clitoris, vaginal area, and anal area; there are also two-pronged vibrators for simultaneous clitoral and anal stimulation. You can buy vibrating butt plugs, which add vibration to all the other features discussed in the previous section, as well as various attachments and sleeves that fit on standard-size vibrators to transform them into anal toys. Vibrators are also great for anal penetration, and vibration can actually relax the anal sphincters. Just make sure that the vibrator is long enough for penetration—over seven inches—and has a flared base. Some men especially enjoy being anally penetrated with a vibrator since vibrators are great for stimulating the prostate gland.

Dildos

I like to fuck a man with a big black dildo.

I love it when my female partner fucks me with her strap-on dildo.

Dildos come in so many different shapes and sizes that there is one for practically every individual taste, need, and desire. There are dildos that look like penises (with balls and realistic-looking heads), dildos that look like torpedoes, and even dildos that look like dolphins. Dildos are made of silicone, latex, or vinyl. Silicone toys tend to be more flexible, smooth, and nonporous, so they're easy to clean. Latex or vinyl is less resilient than silicone but still relatively nonporous. Jellylike dildos (and butt plugs) are very porous and should always be used with a condom. Dildos that curve up from the base (instead of being straight) are often better suited to anal intercourse because they nicely mirror the curve of the rectum. Dildos are the best tools for in-and-out penetration.

For a woman who wants to experience anal penetration with a male partner whose penis is either too big or too long for comfort, dildos provide a great alternative. (A less common scenario is a woman whose partner's penis is not big enough, in which case a dildo can give a girl what she needs). Likewise, for a man who likes to be penetrated by something other than his female partner's fingers, or who wants to experience "being fucked up the ass with a cock," a woman can strap a dildo between her legs and satisfy that desire.

I'm more of a finger/tongue person. But I did once strap on a dildo and do my boyfriend from behind. It was fun but a little awkward because I am shorter than him so I couldn't really reach his head to kiss him. I love the response of my partner [when I am fucking his ass], it gets me more excited. And I like the notion of penetrating someone else's body.

Many women who have sex with other women also like to use dildos to penetrate their partners. Women can experiment with a variety of sizes to find which one is most comfortable. Dildos can give that full feeling as well as satisfy the craving to fuck and be fucked.

Some people like to penetrate their partner with a dildo held in their hand; this tends to give the active partner more control of the dildo and its movement. Others opt to wear a dildo in a harness and have their hands free for other activities. Most harnesses are designed to have the dildo rest in place between one's legs. While lots of women love to fuck this way, a word to novices: like just about everything else, it takes practice. So, for all you guys out there who are thrilled at the idea of a girl with a dick doing you, have some patience while she practices her technique; remember the first time you used that tool of yours, and give her a break while she figures hers out. And for all women fucking with dildos, make sure you talk to your partner, ask what she or he likes, and try different positions to see what works best for both of you. There is also a harness on the market that you strap to your thigh; many women find the thigh harness a great alternative, giving them better flexibility and control of a dildo. The thigh harness is also a way to rectify a significant difference in height or size between two partners.

Anal Beads

Anal beads are latex or plastic beads on a string made of nylon (or sometimes cotton) with a ring on the end. The beads can be the size of marbles all the way up to the size of golf balls. The most popular beads are usually one-half to one inch in diameter. Regardless of their size, make sure the balls are clean, smooth (file the edges if they're not), and well-lubricated and that the string is at least seven inches long. You can also put a condom over the beads and knot the open end of the condom. Cotton strings are much harder to keep clean than nylon; likewise, beads made of soft rubber or jelly rubber are very porous and difficult to disinfect. So most people will want to make sure they get nylon strings and latex beads, or definitely use a condom every time.

Many people like to insert the beads in the rectum while having their genitals stimulated. You should insert one bead at a time, giving the rectum a chance to adjust to the sensation; plus, it can be quite intense to feel the anus contract around each bead. If you've been practicing your Kegel and pelvic exercises, you'll be more aware of these contractions and even be able to control them voluntarily. Some people like to feed the balls inside and then pull them out just as they are climaxing; others like to climax with the beads in and then remove them. Remember to withdraw the beads slowly and gently—pulling the entire string of beads out in one motion too quickly could be uncomfortable.

One final reminder on the subject of beads and balls: you should never put any round objects—marbles, super balls, ping-pong balls, golf balls, ben-wa balls, or any other kind of balls—in your rectum. Besides irritating your rectal tissue, they can also become irretrievable without a speedy trip to the emergency room. Use only beads that are on a string and designed for anal play.

Tips

If you are considering putting something in your anus or someone else's, make sure you use common sense. For best results, make sure the tools and toys you use for anal sex are

- Smooth: Never put any sharp object or anything with rough or jagged edges in the rectum. *Never* put anything glass or breakable in the anus. Even objects made for anal penetration must be smooth; you can file rough edges on dildos or plugs with a regular nail file, and for added smoothness, use a condom.

- Flexible: Make sure that your tool is flexible enough to maneuver those curves in the rectum. Very hard, rigid things (like candles or metal or wooden objects) are not a good idea to insert in your rectum.

- Clean: Make sure that all tools are cleaned with sex toy cleaner or antibacterial soap and hot water; alternatively, you can put a new condom on each tool before using it. Soak toys for about fifteen minutes to disinfect them with Betadine, hydrogen peroxide (full strength), diluted bleach (one part bleach, ten parts water), or a sex toy cleaner.

- Retrievable: Never put anything in a rectum that may get "lost" or will be difficult to retrieve. Make sure plugs have flared bases and that dildos and vibrators are long enough so that the person using them has a good grip.

- Realistic: It's not a good idea to put something of an unrealistic width, length, shape, or size in someone else's or your own anus. Be sensible.

EXERCISE: Window Shopping

It may be helpful for you to get a look at all the toys covered in this chapter in the flesh (so to speak). The exact execution of this exercise depends on where you live. If you live in a town with a sex toy store, a condom store (like Condomania), an adult novelty shop, or an adult video store that carries sex toys, make a date with yourself to go and spend a little time there. Just look at what's available—the different kinds of lubricants, condoms, latex gloves, and so on. If you're interested in exploring anal penetration, peruse the butt plugs, vibrators, anal beads, dildos, and harnesses. If you don't live near such a store, order a mail-order catalog and do a little "window shopping." Some mail-order sources for sex toys have elaborate Web sites, with color images of products and detailed product descriptions. The Shopping Guide (see Resources at the end of this book) lists retailers throughout the United States and Canada who carry a full line of anal toys and sex supplies. Some of these especially cater to women.

NOTES

1. For more information on the Reality™ Female Condom, see the Northwest AIDS Foundation brochure reprinted on the Society for Human Sexuality Web site (see Resources for Web address).

2. McIlvenna, *Complete Guide to Safer Sex*, 82.

3. McIlvenna, *Complete Guide to Safer Sex*, 211.

QUOTES AND SIDEBARS

Cathy Winks and Anne Semans, *The New Good Vibrations Guide to Sex* (San Francisco: Cleis Press, 1997), 163.

Dorian Key, "Every Boy" in *Best Lesbian Erotica 1998* edited by Tristan Taormino (San Francisco: Cleis Press, 1998).

Shaving and Enemas:

Spring Cleaning and Then Some

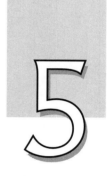

Enemas

So you want to have an enema. First, I want to reiterate that you don't have to have an enema in order to have relatively safe and clean anal sex. Some people find that an enema helps reassure them about the cleanliness of their anuses and the emptiness of their bowels. Others like to give or receive enemas as part of an erotic encounter or an S/M scene; for them an enema does not necessarily go hand in hand with anal sex but becomes an erotic activity unto itself.

When I use the term *enema*, I am referring to a douche of the anal canal and rectum. There are other practices that some people also call enemas—including colonics, high colonics, or cleaning of the transverse colon—which I do not cover in this book.

I cannot stress enough that giving enemas is a skill that takes practice and patience. Your first enema may feel strange. Since your rectum is used to expelling matter, having water flow into it can feel a little weird at first. Don't worry—this sensation of fullness in your rectum just takes some getting used to. When you have a bowel

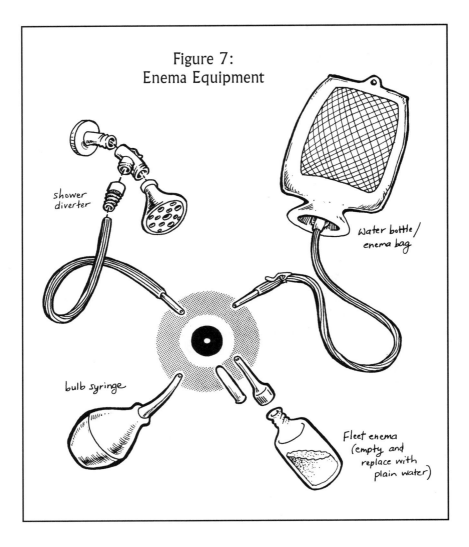

Figure 7:
Enema Equipment

shower diverter

water bottle / enema bag

bulb syringe

Fleet enema (empty and replace with plain water)

movement from an enema, it may feel like having diarrhea. Just remember to listen to your body—an enema can feel different, but it should not be uncomfortable or painful at all.

There are three different kinds of enemas, and I will review them from simplest to most complex (also see figure 7).

Bulb Syringe Enemas

You can purchase a bulb syringe at most drug stores. If you don't want to use a bulb syringe, you can buy an enema kit at a drug store, empty out the chemical solution, and refill the nozzle-tipped bottle with plain warm water.

Many people find that filling a bath with warm water (around 100°F) is the easiest way to begin this kind of enema. Fill the syringe with water and gently insert the tip into your rectum. Lubricate the tip and your anus with water-based lubricant before insertion. Squeeze the bulb to release the water into your rectum. Withdraw the syringe as you continue squeezing, then refill it with water and repeat. Do it a few times or until you feel "full" of water. Wait a few minutes, then get out of the tub, go sit on the toilet, and let nature take its course. You can get back in the tub and repeat the enema (about two to three times) until your bowels are completely cleaned out.

Enema Bag/Hot Water Bottle Enemas

Giving yourself an enema with an enema bag and plastic tubing (also called a fountain syringe) takes a little more skill, and maybe even an assistant. You need an enema bag (which resembles a hot water bottle with a nozzle on the bottom), tubing, and a hook of some kind to hang the bag on (over either the toilet or the tub).

*T*HEN SOMETHING SMALL AND HARD ENTERED HER *anus and forced its way deep as she gave a little gasp, pressing her lips tightly together. Her muscles contracted to fight the little invasion, but this only sent ripples of pleasure through her. The flush of water into her vagina had stopped. And what happened now was unmistakable: A stream of warm water was being pumped into her rectum...It filled her with ever-increasing force, and a strong hand pressed her buttocks together as if bidding her not to release the water.*

It seemed a whole new region of her body came to life, a part of her that had never been punished or even really examined. The force of the flow grew stronger and stronger. Her mind protested that she could not be invaded in this final way, that she could not be rendered so helpless.

She felt she would burst if she did not let go...

She squeezed her eyes shut. She felt warm water poured over her private parts, front and back, heard the loud full rush in the basin.

"Yes, to be purified," she thought. And she experienced a great undeniable relief, the awareness of her body cleansing itself becoming exquisite as she shuddered.

— *ANNE RICE*

Fill the bag with warm water (100°F). Hang the bag within easy reach and no more than eighteen inches above your butt. Find a position that's comfortable; you may want to try lying on your left side with your right leg pulled up to your chest or kneeling with your ass up, your head down, and one side of your face against the floor. Again, apply some water-based lubricant to the tip of the nozzle and inside your anus. Gently insert the tube into your rectum, then release the valve on the bag until water begins to flow at the desired pressure (very low pressure is best). You'll know when you've had enough. When you feel full, close the gauge, take the tube out, and go to the toilet. Repeat several times until only water comes out during a bowel movement.

Shower Attachment Enemas

You can buy an attachment for your shower—called the aluminum nozzle attachment, the silver bullet attachment, or the shower bidet attachment—through sex shops or mail-order catalogs. After you've attached it to your shower, set the temperature to a comfortable level of warmth and the flow to a desired speed and pressure (slower is better, especially for beginners). Again, find a comfortable position, like kneeling, squatting, or standing with one leg up on the edge of the tub. Slip the tube inside, take as much water as you can, and hold it for a few minutes. If you have an exceptional drainage system, you may want to remain in the shower and shoot the water back out. Doing it right in the shower means you don't have to keep jumping in and out, and the mess will wash right down the drain. Or you can return to the toilet to ensure less mess. Repeat the enema until you're all clean, usually two or three times total—*don't overdo it.*

General Tips for a Safe Enema

- You should feel no discomfort during an enema; if you experience pain or cramping, go sit on the toilet right away.
- If you're having an enema in preparation for anal sex, you should do it at least two to three hours prior to having sex to give your body a chance to reabsorb water and recover.
- Storebought enemas like the Fleet Ready-to-Use Enema™ contain laxatives and harsh chemicals that can irritate your rectum; plain filtered water without additives is a better idea. Never use a vaginal douche in your rectum.
- Do not use a turkey baster to give yourself or your partner an enema. Turkey basters are too long and are made of plastic that is inflexible and may have rough seams.
- Depending on the state of your water supply, you may want to use heated bottled water (100°F).
- I've heard about vodka enemas, coffee enemas, and other exotic enemas, but these are really not good for you. Any liquid you put in your rectum gets absorbed so quickly that it's like shooting it in your veins. It will ultimately irritate your rectum, and it could make you very, very sick.
- Allow yourself plenty of time and several bowel movements before you're cleaned out.
- Do not share enema equipment.
- Clean and disinfect your enema equipment carefully (diluted liquid bleach is a good disinfectant).
- Carefully read and follow all instructions that accompany enema kits or equipment.
- It's not a good idea to have enemas too frequently. They tend to stress out your rectum, and too much of this evacuation can throw your rectum, bowels, and

gastrointestinal tract off balance. According to sex educator Robert Morgan, frequent use of enemas can wash away mucosa from your rectum and cause colitis/proctitis.

• If, after an enema, you don't have a bowel movement or expel any liquid, you could be dehydrated or have a serious condition. See a doctor immediately.[1]

The Barber and the Back Door: Shaving the Anal Area

Although it is not widely discussed, many people find that shaving their own or their partner's anal area can be very erotic. Guidelines for shaving the anal area are very similar to those for shaving a woman's pubic area or a man's balls and pubic area. Use a regular disposable razor—leave the wielding of straight razors to the professionals—and plenty of nonirritating shaving cream (I find Aveeno Shaving Gel™ with oatmeal ideal). Find a clean, well-lit place to work, go slowly, and be careful. If you're shaving your own anus, use a hand-held mirror so you can see exactly what you're doing.

It's probably a good idea not to shave the anal area right before you're planning to have sex; since you'll have a greater chance of having nicks or cuts, be extra careful and definitely practice safer sex. One more thing: when the hair grows back, it will itch, so use a soothing lotion.

NOTES
1. For more information on enemas, I recommend you read Bert Herrman, *Trust: The Hand Book (A Guide to the Sensual and Spiritual Art of Handballing)* (San Francisco: Alamo Square Press, 1991).

SIDEBAR
Anne Rice, "Beauty: The Rites of Purification," from *Beauty's Release* by Anne Rice, writing as A. N. Roquelaure (New York: Plume, 1985), 53–54.

Doing It For Yourself:

Masturbation and Anal Eroticism

I remember being about eight or nine and while masturbating inserting the handle of a paintbrush (the closest phallic object at hand) in my ass... I had just read somewhere that this was pleasurable and was curious. It was.

The best introduction to anal eroticism starts with your own behind. In the 1970s, consciousness-raising groups spawned by the women's movement encouraged women to explore their vaginas and do gynecological self-examination with a speculum to gain a better understanding of their bodies; the more knowledge women have about our own bodies, the more in touch we can be with our gynecological health as well as our sexual pleasure. But many of us are not familiar with how our own anuses look and feel; we are taught to think of them as private, dirty, and absolutely not a source of pleasure.

Since most of us

struggle with periods of

self-hatred, bad body

images, shame and

confusion over

sex and pleasure,

I recommend having a

hot love affair with

yourself. Sexual healing

begins by learning how

to turn yourself on,

discovering your sexual

fantasies, and giving

yourself an abundance

of selflove and orgasms.

—*Betty Dodson*

Unlike men, who only have to glance down to see one important source of their libido, women have to find a well-lit room, a comfortable position, and a mirror just to see our own vaginas and clitorises. The same is true for our anuses. Looking at your anus, touching it, stroking it, feeling how it responds to even the lightest touch can give you a world of information about anal eroticism. While you're exploring your anal area, you will want to use the preparations outlined in chapter 2: Relax and be patient with yourself. Go slowly in the beginning and don't try to do too much all at once. Make sure you have a big bottle of lubricant nearby in addition to latex gloves and anal toys, if you wish. Do what feels good, and stop if and when it stops feeling good. Also remember that anal stimulation may be something you want to reserve for your "sex for one" occasions, which is fine; there will be plenty of time to bring anal eroticism to sex with a partner if and when you'd like to do that.

My first experience was as a twelve-year-old. I recall taking a shower and cleaning my genitals and ass. I noticed that the soap running along my anus felt really good, so I slid a finger inside myself and began moving it in and out. Eventually, I got enough manual dexterity to rub my clit with a bar of soap and fuck my anus simultaneously.

In addition to being fun, exciting, and arousing, exploring anal eroticism during masturbation is also the best way to prepare for anal sex with a partner. If you want to have your anus penetrated by your partner, exploring it by yourself will help you figure out what you enjoy and what you don't. Experiencing anal pleasure by yourself can also help to reassure you that it can be pleasurable with a partner; you'll know what it feels like when it feels good. Your own exploration can also serve to get your anus used to stimulation and penetration. If the first finger that slips in your anus is your own, then someone else's won't seem so scary and may even feel better than you had imagined!

Be sweet to your little "rosebud."

—*Betty Dodson*

If you want to penetrate someone else's anus, exploring your own anal area by yourself will give you insight into what's going on down there, including the ins and outs of the anus, anal canal, and rectum: the sensitive tissue, the all-important curves of the rectum, and the various sensations of anal stimulation and penetration. Self-pleasuring your anus will give you a good sense of what your partner might feel as you give him or her pleasure. I believe the best way to become skilled at doing something to someone else is to practice it on yourself first.

Remember, because of the contractions the anal sphincters can make during arousal and climax, the anus can actually "suck" objects into it. There won't be anyone else in the room to prevent a toy from going too far inside your rectum. It is crucial that anything you put in your anus besides your finger have a flared base.

When you're ready to explore anal eroticism during masturbation, you might want to begin by taking a warm, leisurely bath or shower. The bath or shower will help you relax as well as give you an opportunity to get your anus nice and clean and ready for fun. Also make sure your hands are clean and your nails are trimmed neatly. Begin by masturbating as you usually do; start by doing what you know first, which for most of us will mean stimulating the vagina and clitoris. Bring out that favorite vibrator or dildo, turn on a hot porn video or a steamy movie— do whatever will get you aroused. Don't jump right into exploring your anus; instead, simply masturbate and get your entire body aroused.

When you feel juiced up and ready to pay some attention to your anal area, you may want to use a mirror so you can see exactly what's going on down there. Find a comfortable position. Lying on your back or sitting in a comfy chair or on the edge of the bed might be best at first so you can look in a mirror. If you've already practiced with a mirror or aren't using the mirror, you can lie on your stomach, lie on your side, or stand up (perhaps in the shower); find a position that works for you, one that allows you to stimulate your clitoris and reach your anus.

I usually masturbate on my stomach; that is the most familiar position for me and the one in which I get most easily aroused. When I began exploring anal eroticism during masturbation, I found it easy to begin on my stomach, then turn over on my back so I could look at my butt in the mirror.

Begin with some relaxation techniques like deep breathing or meditation; you may also want to do some Kegel exercises to get warmed up and get the blood flowing to your anus. Gently massage your buttocks, your inner thighs, and the area around your anus. Note how the opening responds to the massage around it. Put on a latex glove (if you want to) and pour some lubricant into your hand. Make sure your finger is good and slippery.

When you feel comfortable, gently touch your anus. Stroke it, rub it, let the lube glide over your skin. Just stimulating the opening can be extremely pleasurable because of all the nerve endings in the anal area. You may also want to use a vibrator to stimulate the outside of your anus; vibrations can both relax the area and get the blood pumping there. Spend time feeling your way around and exploring how your whole body responds to your anus being stroked, rubbed, played with, and teased. A good next step is to use your finger to press gently at the opening. Feel how your body responds to the pressure against your anal opening. Keep touching and pressing until you feel ready for more. You may want to continue to stimulate your clitoris to get further aroused; remember, masturbating gets the whole pelvic area stimulated and engorged.

Continue by adding more lube to your finger and inserting just the tip into your anus; stay there and let yourself get used to the feeling. Add some lubricant. Move your finger gently against the sides of the opening without going any farther inside. When you feel ready, venture a little farther. See how the sphincter muscles feel around your finger. You may want to continue to masturbate with your other hand or use a vibrator. Remember to be patient with yourself, go at your own pace, and listen to your body. If at any time you feel discomfort or pain, stop. There's no rush. Keep nudging the finger inside until it's as far as you want it to go.

Experiment with all the different sensations you can create with just one finger. You can try a slow probe, venturing inside inch by inch, experimenting with a variety of depths. Some people like a circular motion, creating circles just inside the anus with a finger and feeling the walls of the anus contracting around the finger. Other people enjoy the feeling of simply having something in their anus; see what it feels like to rub your clitoris while your finger stays still in your anus. You can also practice some in-and-out play, trying different speeds and rhythms as you slide your finger in and out of your anus. Savor each new movement and sensation.

As you get more experienced, you can repeat this exercise with more lube and more fingers. When you can comfortably fit about two fingers inside, you may want to graduate to a slim butt plug, dildo, or vibrator. Remember, plugs are good for that full feeling, dildos for in-and-out action, and vibrators for in-and-out and, of course, vibration. Because these toys are longer than your fingers, you can use them to probe more deeply into the rectum. Make sure to use plenty of lube and start out slowly. Pay attention to how the muscles contract around the toy; make sure to let your anus get used to the feeling each time you inch a little farther inside. You'll notice a difference as your tool moves from the anal canal into the rectum. In the anus, you'll experience more resistance and a tighter feeling. In the rectum, you will feel like there's more room.

If you rush penetration, your anus is likely to get sore and you'll have to stop all activities before you might want to. If you listen to your body and give your anus a chance to get fully aroused, it will open up and give you plenty of room for penetration by a slim dildo and, eventually, even bigger things.

SIDEBARS
Betty Dodson, *Sex for One: The Joy of Selfloving* (New York: Three Rivers Press), 157, 143. Author and sex educator Betty Dodson is considered by many to be the "mother of masturbation."

Let Your Tongue Do the Walking

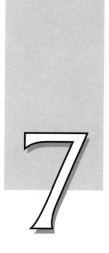

Analingus

Analingus, known more commonly as "rimming," is stimulation of the anal area with the mouth and tongue—licking, flicking, nibbling, sucking, circling, and tongue-fucking. Many people love the simple pleasure of having their anus licked or licking a partner's anus. Because the anal area is so full of nerve endings, even the tiniest sensations can register high on the turn-on meter.

> I love when my boyfriend has been licking my pussy for a long time, getting me really turned on, then travels down and starts licking around my asshole. The feeling of his tongue lightly flicking against my skin just sends me over the edge!

A good way to introduce rimming is to begin by nibbling and licking your partner's buttocks. As is true for other activities, it's important to explore and pleasure the whole area, rather than diving right into the crown jewel. Once you're ready to put your mouth on the anus, start out slowly.

I use my tongue to explore every little nook of my lover's asshole. Because the hole is puckered, there are a million little folds and crevices to find and lick.

Many people feel especially anxious about rimming because of the association between the anus and defecating; we learn at an early age that if something is dirty or smells bad, we shouldn't put our mouth on it. Remember that there are normally only trace amounts of feces in the anus and anal canal. If you and your partner are especially concerned about cleanliness, your partner could have an enema. (Remember an enema should be done at least two hours before the sexual encounter). Aesthetically speaking, analingus need not be any more dirty or messy than cunnilingus. Some people find the anus disgusting or gross, just as some unenlightened folks find the vagina and clitoris unappealing. Yet many of us approach cunnilingus with desire and enthusiasm and feel the same about analingus. Keep in mind, however, that besides HIV and STDs, we come into contact with trace amounts of feces from the colon, which may carry parasites, hepatitis A, and other viruses.

Let your mouth, lips, and tongue explore your lover's anus freely, and experiment with different techniques as you go along. Listen to your partner's verbal and nonverbal responses and let those help to guide you. Some people like to really thrust their tongues in and out of their partner's anus; you can penetrate your lover's anus to ecstasy.

I really like my asshole licked and sucked, but I don't like penetration with fingers or anything. One time, my lover stuck her tongue inside me and it felt great. So, I guess I do like penetration— but only with someone's tongue.

There are a variety of positions you can try for analingus. Some people like to lick their partner's anus from behind in the "doggie-style" position, with the receiving partner on hands and knees. Others like to create a version of the sixty-nine position, so they can pleasure each other simultaneously. You can lick your partner's anus from almost any position, including standing, sitting, or lying down. Experiment with what is most comfortable and pleasurable for both of you.

> I like to have my lover on her back with a pillow under her butt, her knees bent and legs up in the air. I put one hand on each of her cheeks, and spread them apart. Then, I cover her hole with my tongue and lips, slipping the tip of my tongue just inside her ass.

Rimming can be incredibly pleasurable for everyone involved, including the person giving the pleasure. Nina Hartley demonstrates in her anal sex video:

> Rimming is extremely, extremely pleasurable...
> It's important to keep in mind that if you're performing analingus, give your mouth a good time.
> Again, it's never something that you're just doing to the other person; it's something you're sharing with each other. As happy as my [ass] is, his mouth is equally as happy.[1]

*H*IS CUTE LITTLE PUCKER-KISS OF AN ASSHOLE *comes into view, looking for all the world like it's there for your delectation. You extend your tongue and lick the sweet, tangy little entrance. He groans.*

—LINDA JAIVIN

Analingus and Safer Sex

If you plan to venture around and inside the anus, and you are nonmonogamous, you should definitely practice safer sex by always using a barrier for anal contact. Rimming without a latex barrier is considered a high-risk activity for the transmission of STDs and HIV.

If you are monogamous or fluid-bonded, you may still wish to use a barrier. Some women and their partners choose not to, but be aware of the risks you are taking if you make that choice. Remember, fecal matter in the rectum and anal canal may contain hepatitis A, amoeba, parasites, intestinal viruses—all of which can infect you or your partner and make you sick.

A barrier can be a dental dam (a square of latex usually available where sex toys are sold), plastic wrap (like Saran Wrap), an unlubricated condom cut lengthwise, or a latex glove cut into a usable shape. Dab some lube on the side that covers the anus. Some people like to cut up latex gloves for analingus and cunnilingus because you can use one of the glove's fingers to stick your tongue in (see figure 8).

If you're not using a barrier, rinse thoroughly with mouthwash after rimming before putting your mouth elsewhere (like on someone's vagina or penis) to prevent the spread of bacteria.

NOTES
1. Hartley, *Guide to Anal Sex.*

SIDEBAR
Linda Jaivin, *Eat Me* (New York: Broadway Books/Bantam Doubleday Dell Publishing Group, 1997), 220.

Figure 8:
Making a Dental Dam

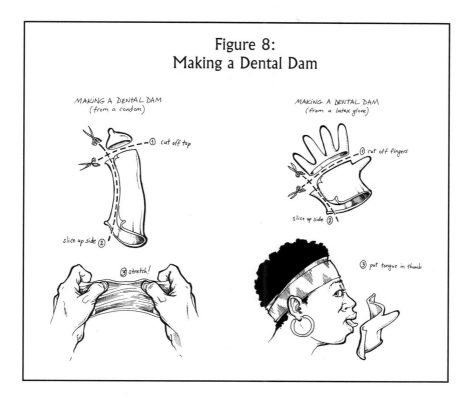

Anal
Penetration

Insertive Anal Penetration

A captain steering a ship through a turbulent
ocean knows that it is the water that is in control;
the captain's job is tuning in and maneuvering
through the tides and currents.[1]

As the insertive partner in anal sex, your job is to go
slowly, be gentle, communicate, progress at a reasonable
pace, and let your partner take control of the ship.

Go Slowly, Be Gentle

*I like to give a long and titillating anal massage
which builds up externally for a long time and
then becomes penetrative with a finger and*

sometimes toys. Where the other person just receives. I also like humping the butt (not penetrative), with the other person face down and me on top of them.

Review the basic preparations, especially the relaxation exercises. Start out with some fun, stress-free foreplay. Getting someone aroused in an overall way will make the transition to anal play easier and smoother. Kiss her on the favorite spot of hers. Stroke that place you know will drive him wild. When your partner is ready to progress to anal stimulation, make the transition slowly. Start out by massaging the buttocks and inner thighs. Work your way around the anal area with your fingers, your mouth, or a vibrator. The more you stimulate the entire area, the more the blood rushes there. You can combine anal stimulation with stimulation of the clitoris, vagina, or penis to get the entire genital region engorged and excited.

*H*E CLAMPS UP TO PREVENT ME FROM RUBBING HERE, *but aggression has risen in me and I press on, massaging a moistened finger at the entrance. It's slick there, and I can imagine the smell, which excites me; I know that he's concerned about the smell, too—how I'll find him—and this excites me. The thought pops into my mind that if I had a dick, right now if I had a dick, I would wear him out..."*

—MAGENTA MICHAELS

For me, it helps to relax my anus if I'm having clitoral stimulation…If it's just my butt, it's like a hot piece of intense sensation. If I put something on my clit like the vibrator, the whole area becomes like a giant clit…Every time you stroke your clit, [your ass] relaxes and opens up.[2]

When your partner is ready for penetration, begin with one well-lubricated finger. Insert only the tip, up to the first knuckle, and stay there. Since the first instinct of the sphincter muscles will be to tighten, let the anus get used to having something inside it and let the sphincter muscles relax. A good way to further relax the receptive partner's anus is to *slowly* and *gently* push up and down against the opening.

I love feeling the tightness of that hole around my fingers, the heat. I love the feeling that I always have to push my way in, like I'm discovering a new hole.

Often, the sphincter muscles of the anal canal will respond to penetration by contracting around the object, then releasing. Many sex educators call this motion "winking." Never poke the anus; instead, stroke the opening with the pad of your finger. If you gently caress the anus, it will wink at you. The anus will open, and you can slowly slide a well-lubricated finger inside.[3]

There are so many nerve endings in the anal area that every sensation is magnified. Keep in mind that a light touch, a slim pinkie, and a slight wiggle all go a long way toward arousing your partner. The simplest caress can be extremely pleasurable. If she wants more, deeper, faster, or harder, she'll tell you. In the beginning, it's best to err on the side of caution and gentleness.

Listen and Talk to Your Partner

It's important that you focus on your partner as you're giving him or her anal pleasure. The receiver should feel comfortable to talk as much as he or she wants during the experience. Ask her how she feels; ask him what he wants. You should also listen to your partner's body. Feel how the sphincter muscles contract around your finger and respond to your touch. Observe the level of tightness and openness of the anus in addition to the rest of the body's response to anal stimulation. What verbal and nonverbal cues is she giving you? How is her breathing pattern? What kinds of sounds is she making? Tell your partner what you're doing, especially each time you are about to move on to something new. Also tell her or him what *you're* feeling, what's turning *you* on; it will enhance the communication and pleasure between you. Ask her to tell you what she likes—does she want more teasing? Some rimming? More pressure and fullness? Less in-and-out motion? Ask her.

> *I like the feel of the power I have when I am inside someone anally. I particularly enjoy this feeling when my partner is face down. I also love to talk sexually about what I am doing anally to someone, like "Boy, you have such a sweet tight ass. Your ass is making my cock very happy..."*

Let Your Partner Take the Lead

The person receiving the anal pleasure should be the one in control. Encourage him or her to breathe deeply; stay where you are on the inhale and nudge farther in on the exhale. Or, instead of you guiding the insertion, the receptive partner can take you inside at her or his pace. As a receiver practices controlling the sphincter muscles, she or he can actually suck you inside.

Make sure your partner knows that if she wants you to stop, she need only say so and you will stop. *Never* coax or pressure a partner into having anal sex. If your partner isn't interested in exploring anal sexuality or isn't in the mood on a particular occasion, respect his or her wishes.

Anal sex can be very highly charged even for the most willing, aroused, or experienced receivers. Having your anus penetrated can be intense, emotional, even a little scary. Keep all these factors in mind, and remember that your partner has put a tremendous amount of trust in you. Respect that trust as well as your partner's body. Realize that she or he may be feeling particularly vulnerable or maybe a little anxious. Reassure your partner that she or he is in charge.

> It is an incredible high to be shown such trust and vulnerability with another person. Here is a part of the body through which we can experience intense pleasure and through which often much damage, shaming, and abuse has been done. Giving gives me a great sense of power. Not the power to hurt, but the power to please, to tease, to entice. And, as a woman, getting to be inside, especially to penetrate a man, is hot and divine. As it should be.

Receptive Anal Penetration

Relax

Relax, relax, relax. Take a deep breath. And another. Relaxation is so important to having pleasurable anal sex; yet I think that with the hectic pace of our lives, it is one of the hardest states to achieve. Because the anus can be a place where we store much of our stress and tension, we need to give our bodies plenty of time to release that tension before venturing into anal pleasure. I find that doing about fifteen minutes of deep breathing helps my body to unwind, and the breathing actually gets me in touch with how my entire body is feeling. A warm bath, candles, and a sensuous massage are also great relaxers. We must also relax our minds, and some people like to meditate or even do some positive visualization to calm and prepare themselves for anal penetration. Ultimately, our bodies and minds are intrinsically linked, and relaxation is a reflexive process.

Tell Your Partner What You Want

You need to figure out what your anal erotic desires are and take responsibility for communicating them to your partner. Although it may seem paradoxical, you *are* the one in the driver's seat. You set the pace and control the action. You need to be well aware of your body, and specifically of your anal sphincters, because you have the ability to relax

HE'S MOVING IN HER, LIGHT AND QUICK, working her ass so sweetly she wants to scream. She's going to come. She stays there a while, riding the knowledge, her clit full and her cunt dripping and her ass on fire. It's so dark with the blindfold, and all she can think about is how good it will be when she comes, how good it will feel, how it doesn't matter about her ass being sore, how nothing matters but this come.

—ROSE WHITE AND ERIC ALBERT

them. Talk to your partner before, during, and after about what turns you on, the sensations you experience, what you'd like more of, and how everything feels.

> It can be alienating for me; it's something I only want to do with people I have an emotional connection with. For me, it is a bit like having sex when I'm drugged: it's extremely intense, a complete giving over to another, but it involves a vulnerability that I only want to enact with someone I love. [I think] "Here is my body: drink," when I am fucked up the ass.

The more information you can give your partner, the better equipped he or she will be to please you. As discussed in chapter 3, it is equally important that your share your fantasies *and* your fears about anal sex. The more in touch you are with your needs, your desires, and your own body, the better the experience will be for everyone.

Take the Lead

Once you are relaxed and ready for penetration, put some lube in your anus and find a position that's comfortable for you. Some people like to be on their back with their legs in the air or on the insertive partner's shoulders; this way, you can face each other, have easier verbal and nonverbal communication, and incorporate other stimulation with anal penetration. Some women like to sit on top of their partners (also facing each other) so they can control the pace and depth of penetration. Many people like to be on all fours, belly down with their butt in the air. This "doggie-style" position can allow better depth and requires the least bending of the rectum. Experiment with various positions until you find what's most comfortable.

Because you are in control of the action, you must be prepared to tell your partner to slow down, change activities, or stop altogether. Listen to your body; if you feel any discomfort or pain, you absolutely need to stop. Don't fool yourself that the pain will subside or pressure yourself to continue even when it no longer feels good. *Anal sex does not have to be uncomfortable or painful at all.*

For Both Partners

Work Your Way Up

If your partner is interested in being penetrated with something bigger than a finger—several fingers, a butt plug, a vibrator, a dildo, or a penis—it's a good idea to set some realistic goals. Set a series of goals that will give both of you room to relax, practice, and feel free from pressure to do too much at once. As penetration progresses, each time you either add a finger or increase the size of the toy, be sure to add more lube and let the anal canal and rectum get used to the new sensation. Just as you let your partner take the lead in the pace, let her or him take the lead in the depth of penetration. Let her ease her anus down onto your fingers or that favorite plug, taking as much as she wants at her pace. You should always begin small and work your way up to big, and remember that you don't have to reach the ultimate goal in one single night.

Once you've worked your way up from fingers to toys or a penis, remember your anatomy lesson and those two curves you're going to run into in the rectum. Each person's rectum is unique, so don't assume that a technique that worked on one person will make your current partner scream in ecstasy. Going slowly will help you navigate the curves of the rectum and begin to discover the individuality of your partner's anal canal and rectum without causing discomfort. There will be plenty of time later for a hard-and-fast frenzy, if that's what you both want. But, in general, you shouldn't make any swift or jerky movements. Likewise, whenever you withdraw anything from the anus—if she asks you to stop, after she's had an orgasm, or when you're going to take a break— always pull out slowly. Even if your partner says "Get it out of me now!" don't withdraw too quickly or you can hurt or tear the tender rectal tissue.

I TAKE HER ASS IN MY TWO HANDS, LIKE A BIG FRUIT, and push it upwards, and while my tongue is playing there in the mouth of her sex, my fingers press into the flesh of her ass, travel around its firmness, into its curve, and my forefinger feels the little mouth of her anus and pushes gently.

Suddenly Mary gives a start—as if I have touched off an electric spark. She moves to enclose my finger. I press it farther, all the while moving my tongue inside of her sex. She begins to moan, to undulate.

When she sinks downwards she feels my flicking finger, when she rises upwards she meets my flicking tongue. With every move, she feels my quickening rhythm, until she has a long spasm and begins to moan like a pigeon. With the finger I feel the palpitation of pleasure, going once, twice, thrice, beating ecstatically.

—ANAÏS NIN

Positions for Anal Penetration

All the positions people employ for vaginal penetration can be used for anal penetration. Since everyone has individual needs, tastes, and desires, it is important to experiment with all kinds of positions to discover what works best for you and your partner.

Missionary Position (figure 9)

Among hip, liberated women, the missionary position has gotten a bad rap in recent years because it works well for men but usually affords women no clitoral stimulation. There are plenty of ways to slightly amend this "traditional" position to make it work for you. This position finds the receptive partner on her or his back and the insertive partner

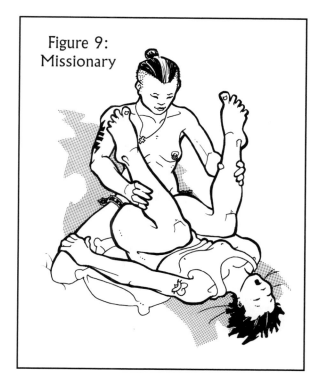

Figure 9: Missionary

on top. Because both partners face each other, it is easier to communicate, especially nonverbally, plus you can attend to other parts of your partner's body— suck on her nipples, kiss his neck, nibble her lips. Many people in the receptive position like missionary-style anal penetration because lying on their back either

feels more comfortable or allows them a sense of sur-
rendering to their partner.

> I like to be on my back when she fucks me in the
> ass. She's in control and I feel like I am giving my
> body over to her. If she uses her hand, she can do
> my butt and work my clit at the same time. If
> she's got the strap-on on, and we get at just the
> right angle, her thrusts can rub my clit.

> When my lover is on her back, I feel like I am top-
> ping her and her ass is mine. It's powerful,
> although I know that she's the one who's really in
> charge.

The receptive partner may find that a pillow under
her butt makes for easier penetration, and she can bend
her knees or either bring her legs to her chest or rest them
on her partner's shoulders. Although the latter position
may create a better angle for entry, it is one that even the
most flexible among us often find hard to sustain. In this
position, your partner usually cannot provide clitoral
stimulation, but you can provide your own with your
hand or a vibrator.

Receptive Partner on Top (figure 10)

In the receptive-partner-on-top position, the receptive
partner can control the angle and depth of penetration.
Straddling the insertive partner, she or he can sit straight
up, or lean forward or backward according to her or his
own desires. Again, facing each other means you can talk
and communicate as well as stroke, rub, pinch, and stimulate other parts of each other's bodies; this position is
also great for clitoral stimulation. Receptive partners can
really take the lead in this position and be in charge of the
depth of insertion, the amount of movement, and the

rhythm of whatever is doing the penetrating—finger(s), butt plug, dildo, or penis.

> I like to be on top for anal sex. I can slowly sit down on his dick, taking my time to make sure my ass is ready. He can play with my clit as I lower myself onto him, and he loves to look at me, and talk dirty to me while we're doing it.

Insertive partners who are inexperienced, nervous about how to penetrate their partners anally, or fearful of hurting their partners may find this position most relaxing because the receiver can do much of the decision making and work. The partners on the bottom often report liking this position best because they get a great view of their partner and can watch them as they receive pleasure.

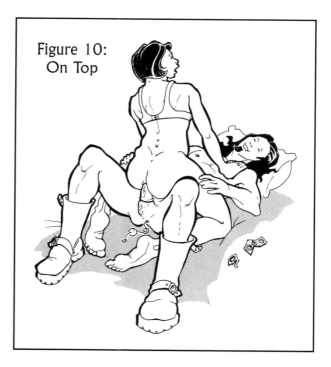

Figure 10: On Top

> If we have anal penetration with the dildo, I want her to be in charge. She knows better how fast and deep to go, plus I like to see her do all the work.

Doggie-Style (figure 11)

The doggie-style position is probably the first one many of us think of when we think about anal sex. Doggie-style is also a popular image in porn magazines and videos. This position, with the receptive partner on her hands and knees and the insertive partner behind her, is best for deep penetration. Because the rectum is in the most straight (not bent) position, the insertive partner can get good depth that is also comfortable to the receiver. If the receptive partner is a woman, this position also makes it easy to reach around and rub her clitoris.

Doing it doggie-style also means both partners can have lots of pelvic movement. The insertive partner can do a lot of deep, hard, or fast thrusting; the receptive partner can move back on or ride fingers, a dildo, or penis from this angle. Many people like to have their partner penetrate them from behind for a fast and frenzied kind of fuck. As when the receptive partner is on top, she can also be in control of the action if the insertive partner does less of the movement and lets the receiver come to her.

I love doggie-style the best. My boyfriend starts out slowly, but as my ass opens up, he can really fuck me from behind just like he fucks my pussy. He says he likes it too because he loves the feeling of my butt cheeks slamming against him.

For giving, I like her on all fours with her ass in the air so I can see all the activity. For receiving— being on all fours or on my back...My favorite of all, though, is being bent over a table and gettin' it from behind.

My current partner can be an incredibly sensual, effeminate submissive male. I love to see him with

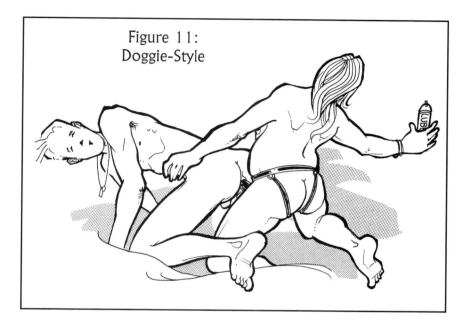

Figure 11:
Doggie-Style

*his ass in the air and his back arched, and I love
the way he looks when I tell him to ride my cock
and he thrusts himself back against me while I just
kneel there, occasionally grabbing his hips or
slapping his butt.*

In a variation on this position, the receptive partner is
on her stomach with her knees either bent or straight.
Although this one may seem awkward on first try, it just
takes a little practice. This, too, is a good position for
medium or deep penetration because the rectum is in an
optimum position for smooth entry (as long as you don't
forget that important curve!).

Spooning and Reverse Spooning (figure 12)

In the spooning position, both partners are on their sides
either facing each other or facing the same direction. This

position is comfortable, flexible, and easily maneuverable, and it gives both partners good control over the angle and depth of penetration; it's an ideal position for partners who are of very different heights or sizes. Some

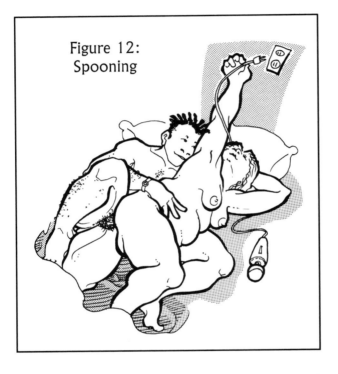

Figure 12:
Spooning

people find that lying side by side gives them greater access to their partner's vagina, clitoris, penis, balls, and other parts of each other's bodies for exploration and stimulation. You don't get the depth of penetration this way that you get with other positions; however, spooning is good for a long, slow anal fucking session, where no one's

in a rush to get somewhere. But don't get me wrong—you can still have ecstatic orgasms this way.

> Side-by-side works for me. She can do my ass and my clit and not go too deep. I like to have her fingers just a little ways into my butt. For me, that's the most sensitive part.

I have gone over the major positions, but I have by no means covered all the possible ones. There are plenty more for you to explore. Some people like to reverse the receptive-partner-on-top position and face the same direction rather than each other. Couples who are similar in size may find they can have anal sex standing up or with one person bent over a bed or table.

I like to be bent over the bed, standing, face down.

I love the feeling of having my partner penetrate me anally and vaginally at the same time using a dildo or vibrator in either orifice. I have often fantasized about having two men fucking me and feeling each other's dicks rubbing against each other through my walls.

Think of each new position as an opportunity to explore different depths, speeds, rhythms, and dynamics; there's lots of erotic territory to find simply by changing your point of view.

NOTES
1. Herrman, *Trust,* 43.
2. Hartley, *Guide to Anal Sex.*
3. Sex educator Robert Morgan.

QUOTES AND SIDEBARS
Magenta Michaels, "Taking Him on a Sunday Afternoon" in *Herotica 2: A Collection of Women's Erotic Fiction* edited by Susie Bright and Joani Blank (San Francisco: Down There Press, 1991), 19.
Rose White and Eric Albert, "She Gets Her Ass Fucked Good" in *Best American Erotica 1997* edited by Susie Bright (New York: Simon & Schuster, 1997), 82.
Anaïs Nin, "Mandra" in *Little Birds* (New York: Harcourt Brace Jovanovich Inc., 1979), 131.

Anal Fisting

Myths About Anal Fisting

Just as there are many myths about anal sex in general, there are several misconceptions about anal fisting (or handballing) in particular. The following are a few of the most common myths.

Myth #1: Fisting is literally what it sounds like it is.

Anal fisting is not exactly what it sounds like—you don't just make a fist and stick it in someone's ass. Fisting is a gradual penetration process of adding finger after finger until you can curve your fingers and comfortably fit your entire hand in someone's rectum. Some people may cringe when they read that, but when done safely and properly, fisting can be an incredibly intense, pleasurable experience for both partners. As Bert Herrman, one of the leading experts on anal fisting, reminds us, "The joy comes from the feeling not the anatomical description." [1]

Myth #2: Only gay men practice anal fisting.

In the late 1960s and 1970s, gay and bisexual men popularized the practice of anal fisting, especially in bathhouses and private parties in major urban areas. It is widely believed that people engaged in fisting for decades before the sexual revolution, but the recorded history of the practice in Western culture dates to the late sixties. (According to sex educator Robert Morgan, fisting has been practiced in China and India for thousands of years.) Like other forms of anal sex, anal fisting has become intrinsically linked with gay men, and only gay men, because particular communities of gay men were widely practicing it. However, while not as common as other forms of anal eroticism, anal fisting is practiced and enjoyed by many women, with both female and male partners.

In her erotic writing of the early 1980s, Pat Califia wrote about anal fisting among lesbians who practiced S/M, and by the early 1990s, Bert Herrman reported that both men *and* women subscribed to *Trust/The Handballing*

*T*WO FINGERS, THEN THREE, *sank into Roxanne's ass. She barely noticed. She was humming along on a smooth road. This was so easy, there was so little friction that it barely qualified as fucking. Nevertheless, there was pleasure, enough to turn her into a squirmy little girl, so bad and dirty that she wanted people to bend her over, pull down her panties, put things up her ass, move them in and out, make her tell them how much she liked it and squeal for more.*

—PAT CALIFIA

Newsletter. Some women, in fact, become aware of and interested in anal fisting through gay male pornography. Many women, especially lesbians, enjoy gay male erotic stories, photography, and videos and have learned about techniques and safety from these sources as well as from gay men who practice anal fisting.

> My most erotic fantasies have always revolved around gay male pornographic images, which is part of why anal fisting appeals to me.

Myth #3: Anal fisting is dangerous.

Some people think that anal fisting will leave the receptive partner in diapers or the insertive partner with a disease. When anal fisting is done with patience and care, it will not injure either of you. Insertive partners can practice safer sex to protect themselves from contracting an STD or other diseases. Contrary to some popular misconceptions, being anally fisted will not make you bleed excessively, damage your rectum, stretch out your anus, or rupture your intestines—if done correctly.

Anal Fisting and Safer Sex

Unless you are monogamous or fluid-bonded, you should practice safer sex every time you engage in anal fisting. There are some specific differences between the regular safer sex practices already outlined in the book and the precautions you should take for anal fisting.

Just as you can use water-based lubricants for anal penetration, you can use larger amounts of thicker, water-based lubricants for fisting; however, most experienced fisting aficionados say they prefer oil-based lubes because they are thicker and dry up much less quickly than their water-based counterparts. While you should never use oil-based lubes for vaginal penetration, because they will not naturally flush out of the vagina, they do flush out of the rectum easily during defecation. It is important to remember, however, that you won't be able to use condoms for anal penetration one to two days after oil-based lubricants are used in the rectum, because the oils will destroy latex condoms.

Many fisters use Crisco regularly because it's thick, it's inexpensive, and it works. Regular, rather than butter or other flavors, is recommended. Remember that sticking your hand in a can of Crisco will leave that can full of bacteria and not usable with any new partner. Try Crisco sticks (individually wrapped portions that resemble sticks of butter) or scoop smaller amounts of Crisco out of the can into a separate container for use with one partner and one session; make sure to clean these containers frequently.

If you are nonmonogamous, you should *always* use protective gloves for fisting; the risks that are present for anal penetration are magnified for anal fisting. Bert Herrman outlines these risks for the insertive partner:

> The inside of one's body provides ideal transfer conditions for all sorts of microorganisms including the HIV virus. Surface abrasions in the walls of the large intestines (colon) are an ordinary occurrence even in normal conditions. No matter how clean one gets, one's insides will not be sterile...Minor paper cuts, scratches, and sores on your hands cannot be avoided. Microorganisms can even enter the system at the base of the fingernails.[2]

Latex gloves protect the person doing the fisting as well as the person being fisted. Even monogamous and fluid-bonded partners may prefer using gloves since the rectum is easily irritated by fingernails or rough skin.

While it is a proven fact that vegetable shortening and oil-based lubricants break down latex condoms, latex gloves tend to be much thicker than condoms and therefore can be used for fisting. Many sex educators recommend that you change into a fresh pair of gloves every fifteen to twenty minutes to ensure safety by preventing tiny holes from forming in the latex.

Latex gloves are sold in many drug stores, in bags of small quantities or boxes of fifty or one hundred. Some gloves are certified sterile, others aren't; however, the place you'll be putting your hand won't be sterile (not even with the most fastidious enema), so the gloves do not necessarily need to be sterile. Some gloves are powdered on the inside to make it easier to put them on. You should rinse gloves out because the powder may irritate your partner's delicate, sensitive anal tissue. Herrman has another tip for the glove wearer:

> We also suggest that tops (especially those who are HIV negative) should rub nonoxynol-9...on their hand before inserting into the glove, in the event of leakage. While [nonoxynol-9] effectively kills the HIV virus, tests have shown that [it is] also very irritating to the kind of cells that line the rectum and vagina. This means that nonoxynol-9 may allow the virus to more effectively penetrate faster. So limit this stuff to inside the glove.[3]

Some people wear two gloves or purchase heavier rubber gloves commonly used for household work; these gloves also tend to be longer (more like "opera length"), which can be a plus for people who want to venture beyond the wrist. Keep in mind that heavier gloves tend to decrease the inserter's sensitivity and sense of how lubricated the glove is.

Recently, many people who regularly use latex gloves—especially those in health care professions—have become either allergic to latex or latex-sensitive. If you are sensitive to latex, you might not want to try Herrman's technique of putting nonoxynol-9 inside the glove; you may also want to try well-fitting vinyl gloves. You might try coating your hand with liquid silicone (found in medical supply or auto supply stores) before putting on a latex glove.[4]

Anal Fisting: The How-To's

People who enjoy being penetrated by larger plugs and dildos and like the feeling of fullness and pressure may also delight in being fisted. Fisting takes a *large* amount of everything that anal sex requires: latex, lube, desire, patience, relaxation, communication, and trust. Fisting takes a great deal of time and skill; you should proceed to fisting only after you have become comfortable with extensive anal penetration.

Preparation

In order to prepare yourself to be fisted, it's a good idea to do some Kegel exercises for several weeks beforehand. Get used to contracting and relaxing your anal sphincter muscles. Relax. Deep breathing during foreplay and fisting is a great way to relax, get focused, and get in touch with your body.

I cannot stress enough that a proper diet with enough fiber is a key component to enjoying anal pleasure. Diet is very important for a person who's going to be fisted.

Most people who practice anal fisting recommend an enema for the receptive partner because of the depth of penetration. Chapter 5 covers different types of enemas and how to give them. Remember to have an enema at least two hours before the sexual encounter, avoid using harsh chemical enemas, and don't have enemas too often. An enema clears out not only the "bad" bacteria, but also the "good" bacteria that normally live in and help our digestive systems; you can take acidophilus (available at most health food stores) to bring your system back in balance. Bert Herrman recommends that you eat easy-to-digest food for nineteen to thirty-six hours before your enema, and very little eighteen hours before fisting. Avoid foods containing small seeds (like strawberries).

Some advice before you make a hellish trip to the laundromat: There is going to be some mess, so you should have lots of paper towels on hand. You should also know that oil-based lubricants and anal secretions are not exactly the easiest laundry job. Many fans of fisting recommend using "chucks," plastic sheets used as under-

---

*S*HE PUSHED. *A RIPPLE DESCENDED FROM BEHIND HER breast bone, amplified, became a wave of desperate hard contractions. Kay had a grim, fixed smile on her face. She hung on to Roxanne's thigh with one hand and kept the other one wedged firmly in her asshole. Her rectum opened, closed, opened wider, and Kay slid in. Her querulous asshole flattened out and disappeared. It felt as if her body had swallowed the advancing hand, sucked it in instead of struggling to repel it. Now it was folded up neatly inside her, a miracle, no pain at all, just the gift, the blessing of someone entering and pleasuring this forbidden part of her body. Kay had made this new channel, made it part of her just by touching it. Her lungs hurt. Had she been shouting?*

—*Pat Califia*

pads in hospitals. They are made to absorb, and they are disposable. You can find them at hospital supply stores.

Fisting Techniques and Tips

After the enema, an erotic fisting session should begin like any erotic encounter involving anal penetration. Relax. Do whatever you need to—baths, candles, music, meditation, visualization, deep breathing, massage—to relax each other. Take your time. Focus on your desire for each other, on communicating, and on trusting each other.

You should also experiment with positions. You want to find one that is comfortable for both of you and that allows the easiest entry and depth of penetration. Some people like to be on their backs with their legs on their partner's shoulders. Some like to be in the doggie-style position on hands and knees, affording a good angle of entry.

Others like to be in a sling—a specially designed seat made of leather, canvas, or plastic webbing (like a hammock for one). A sling is usually suspended from the ceiling or a hook high on the wall. You can lie in it comfortably with your head above your waist, and your partner can have good, flexible access to your ass. Slings can be an expensive item at specialty sex and leather stores and are usually purchased by advanced players.

Just as outlined in the techniques for anal penetration, you should work your way up from external stimulation to actual penetration, with all the necessary steps in between. Remember that the initial opening-up process takes time for the receiver. You may want to start with fingers, graduate to a small butt plug, maybe a dildo, then go back to fingers. Or you can use only your hand the entire time. Rather than pushing your way in, let your partner suck your hand inside and guide you to each new level. Work your fingers inside, adding more lubricant as you go, until you have worked up to four fingers.

A good way to begin the handballing process is to put your fingers together to create a point with your hand, and gently slide inside. Stop as soon as you feel resistance and stay there, letting the muscles get used to the feeling. Each person likes a different method for entry. Some people like to move with a slow, constant pressure. Others use a twisting motion to work their way inside. Some let the receiver draw the hand inside or go slowly in and out as you would with a penis or dildo. Some keep their fingers together in the point until they feel like they can spread their fingers slightly. You can also cup your hand with your fingers curled into your palm. The trickiest part of handballing is the first move into the rectum. Make sure that you are well lubed, because this will be a crucial step.

As with each progression of penetration, when you've gotten your hand inside the rectum, stay there for a while. Let your hand get used to the feelings, and let your partner get used to the feelings she or he is experiencing. Now, remember your anatomy lesson and that all-important curve of the rectum. Feel your way as you venture, and let your partner guide your hand. Go as far as feels comfortable for your partner. You don't have to keep going and going; get to a place that feels good, and decide that's as far as you'll go.

Once you're in the rectum, some partners may like you to stay where you are, while you stimulate their genital area with your free hand or a vibrator. Other folks may like some actual in-and-out movement; keep in mind that your movement while fisting should never be too drastic or jerky. Again, it's all about communication between the two of you.

> The challenge is not learning to stretch the anal canal; rather, it is learning to relax and let go, to allow these muscles to accept entrance from the outside with the same ease they should be allowing release from the inside.[5]

If you are the receptive partner, remember that you are in control of the action. It's critical that you pay attention to your body, know your limits, and communicate with your partner. She will take all her cues from you, and so you need to be aware of your desires, your needs, and the sensations you are feeling. Do not push yourself to do something if your body isn't ready. Rest and take a break if you need one. Stop if and when you need to stop. If you listen to your body, when it is ready to take an entire hand inside your rectum, the feeling will be nothing but pleasurable, intense, and ecstatic.

Afterward, you may feel like having another enema in order to clean out all the lubricant. *Do not have an enema.* Your system has been worked over, and an enema will only irritate your rectum, especially if there are minute abrasions. It is a good idea for you to eat and drink something.

You may experience some soreness, gas pain, irregular bowel movements, or slight spotting of blood when you wipe yourself. All this should correct itself within twenty-four hours. Use common sense: if you are bleeding, experiencing severe pain, have a fever, or feel very sick, go see a doctor immediately. But if you've listened to your body, and your partner has listened to you, anal fisting will leave you satisfied and happily exhausted.

NOTES
1. Herrman, *Trust,* 17.
2. Herrman, *Trust,* 22–23.
3. Herrman, *Trust,* 27.
4. Sex educator Robert Morgan.
5. Herrman, *Trust,* 61.

SIDEBAR
Pat Califia, "The Calyx of Isis" in *Macho Sluts* (Los Angeles: Alyson Publications, 1988), 132, 135.

S/M and Genderplay

S/M and Anal Sex

Sadomasochism (S/M) is often misrepresented and misunderstood in mainstream culture; frequently, S/M is equated with whips and chains, violent abuse, and deviant behavior. In reality, S/M has nothing to do with abuse or force—it is a consensual exchange of power arousing to both partners that may or may not involve genital sex. S/M includes one partner who is referred to as the *dominant* or the *top*; this person is in charge of the encounter, or scene, taking an active role in directing the activities. The other partner, referred to as the *submissive* or the *bottom*, takes a receptive role in the scene. Both partners negotiate a scene beforehand, communicating their likes and dislikes as well as their physical and emotional boundaries and limits.

S/M encompasses a broad spectrum of practices, including but not limited to role-playing; dominance and

submission; bondage and discipline; flagellation (spanking, slapping, paddling, whipping); sensory deprivation
with the use of blindfolds, hoods, gags, and/or ear plugs;
and body modification (permanent and nonpermanent
piercing, cutting, branding).[1]

> One of my current fantasies has my partner com-
> ing home while I am scrubbing the floor on my
> hands and knees in a maid's outfit. She puts
> down her bag and tells me not to turn around,
> and then I realize that she is already wearing her
> strap-on as she proceeds to fuck me in the ass.
> HARD.

Anal sex can be a very hot part of an S/M scene for
many different reasons. Because it is already considered
taboo, naughty, and forbidden, those attitudes can be
exaggerated and played with in the context of an erotic
encounter.

> My favorite way to combine S/M and anal play is
> to make her submit to it and then tell her what a
> bad girl she is for wanting it.

*I COULDN'T RESIST RUNNING MY HAND OVER HIS BUM.
He pushed it up into my palm, and I stroked the firm,
muscular globes. I ran my hand lightly down the crack,
past his anus and over his balls. I heard him expel his
breath with a little sigh of pleasure, at which point I
drew myself up and let the lash crack down upon the
beautiful flesh.*

—LINDA JAIVIN

ONLY A SHORT WHILE BEFORE, when she had been kneeling half-naked before René, and Sir Stephen had opened her thighs with both his hands, René had explained to Sir Stephen why O's buttocks were so easily accessible, and why he was so pleased that they had been so prepared: it was because it had occurred to him that Sir Stephen would enjoy having his preferred path constantly at his disposal.

—PAULINE RÉAGE

Sometimes I like to incorporate some of the taboos about ass-fucking into our dialogue during sex, like saying, "Oh, you're such a bad girl—only bad girls like getting it in the ass. How did you get sooooo naughty?"

For men and women interested in relinquishing control, letting someone else decide what goes on, or being told what to do by a top, anal sex provides a perfect activity of surrender. Others find that being anally penetrated is the ultimate experience of submission, yet still very safe because they can set the boundaries and be in control of the action.

I like anal sex because submitting to my partner this way is one of the ultimate gifts I can give her. It is something I crave and absolutely love, but it is also something that takes a great deal of trust for me to do.

S/M can also be an exploration of the limits of your body: how much you can give and take and for how long. Anal play and penetration can be an excellent manifestation of this metaphor.

> It continues to amaze me that it feels really awesome, and that I can take a big butt plug, and that I like it so much. I also like being on the receiving end because...I love the aggressive side that comes out in her when she's fucking me in the ass.

Many people who practice S/M explore the power dynamics of dominance and submission.

> I like the idea of "forced" penetration. The idea of holding my lover down, with a knife to her throat, and forcing myself into her tight ass while verbally humiliating her and pinching her tits and slapping her...I love sensual and nonscene-oriented anal sex, too, but it is...the violation that really gets me off.

For people interested in incorporating anal sex into dominant-submissive role playing, it is especially important to negotiate your desires and boundaries with your partner. Keep in mind that if the mutually agreed upon use of force, bondage, or very hard fucking are involved in a scene with anal play, you should still go slowly and let the receptive partner take the lead. S/M practitioners often explore the edges of pleasure and pain, but these practices should never be conflated with the experience of anal sex. Anal sex should never be forced or painful even in the context of an S/M scene, because you can do damage to your partner's body. When anal sex is consensual and approached with patience, gentleness, and lots of lube, it can be an ecstatic part of S/M play.

Genderplay and Anal Sex

My current partner is a bi woman and we alternately take on different gender roles in our relationship. There is a gender fluidity that is very important to me.

Many people enjoy enacting gender role-playing, "switching" gender roles, or combining gender characteristics during erotic encounters. Genderbending and genderplay are great ways to explore the complexities of our own genders and how they relate to our sexual identities and practices.

Some of the myths associated with anal sex are related to gender and sexual identity, and these make it ripe for genderplay. For example, some men embrace its perceived link to submission and feminization:

I love to be fucked. I fantasize about being a woman. And sometimes about just being a man while my female partner takes on the role of a man in my head. The genderbending and role reversal here can sometimes be threefold as we switch gender, dominance, and identity all at the same time.

Playing with the association between anal sex and gay men, some heterosexual and lesbian couples like to role-play gay male sex scenes:

I like genderplay within anal sex situations…I like to be a "fag" with my (female) partner, who's also a gay man.

With the help of some imagination, sexy dialogue, costumes and props, or a dildo and harness, you and your partner can be just about anyone you want to be.

S HE SPREAD MY LEGS WIDE, *pulled on a latex glove, reached across me to the nightstand for lube, and then began working fingers into my ass. "Don't move your hands," she whispered, while hers invaded me, one long finger at a time, first working in and then starting to fuck—repeating again and again until she had three up my ass and I was as stretched out and full as I'd ever been. Her other hand, ruby ring glinting in the low light from a streetlamp, lay splayed across my belly, holding me down, thumb slowly working my clit, while she fucked my ass with the other. I held the bars but soon writhed crazily with the sensation, and as she fucked me more and more fiercely I raised my legs to her shoulders, spreading my ass as wide to her as I could, wanting to let her get at me as deeply as possible. When she felt my body tighten up in an imminent come, she stopped playing with my clit altogether, pulled my nipple hard, and I orgasmed from her pumping hand alone, coming until I was curled up practically sobbing—but still holding the bars.*

"You're so good!" I gasped when she was finally done with me, and she gave me that small smile again and said, "What I like about assholes is, everybody has one."

—CAROL QUEEN

You can be your girlfriend's boyfriend, your male partner's gay lover, or a "chick with a dick." Your female partner can be a male hustler or your husband. Your male
partner can be a submissive young woman with a strict
mistress or a girly girl being told what to do.

> I absolutely love to penetrate my male partners
> with a strap-on dildo. It's very important to me as
> a newly reformed butch dyke to continue to play
> with gender roles.

Although dildos are not penis replacements, they certainly symbolize a great deal of erotic potential. Women
who strap on a dildo can feel silly, sexy, or wildly powerful:

> Mostly now I have sex with men (actually, I only
> have sex with one man now, but even before that
> it's been mostly men for the past few years), and
> I like to have a penis and fuck with it. I like to run
> around the house with my strap-on on, knowing
> I'm going to use it on my partner, who is nervous
> but excited; it makes me feel silly and selfish and
> rude and excited. I am typically more of a bottom
> in bed, but when I put on my penis, I am über-
> top, with a whole new erotic personality.

Combining genderplay and anal sex is a way to
explore a range of fantasies: enacting a more dominant,
aggressive role; experiencing a submissive, receptive role;
or assuming a different sexual identity altogether. Because
everyone has the anal orifice in common, anal sex can be
both the great equalizer and a source of genderbending,
fantasy, and unlimited erotic possibilities.

NOTES
1. Read more about S/M in *Leatherfolk,* edited by Mark Thompson (Boston: Alyson, 1991); *Coming to Power,* edited by SAMOIS (Boston: Alyson, 1982); *The Second Coming,* edited by Pat Califia and Robin Sweeney (Los Angeles: Alyson, 1996); *Different Loving* by Gloria Brame (Random House, 1993); *Sensuous Magic* by Pat Califia (New York: Masquerade, 1996); *SM 101* by Jay Wiseman (San Francisco: Greenery Press, 1992).

SIDEBARS

Linda Jaivin, *Eat Me* (New York: Broadway Books/Bantam Doubleday Dell Publishing Group, 1997), 164.

Pauline Réage, *Story of O,* translated by Sabine d'Estree (New York: Grove Press, 1965), 83.

Carol Queen, "Ariel" in *The Leatherdaddy and the Femme* (San Francisco: Cleis Press, 1998).

Anal Health

Taking Care of Your Ass

Many people assume that if you regularly engage in anal sex, you are more likely to develop anal ailments. Several common myths perpetuate this idea; myths about receptive anal sex partners getting hemorrhoids or anal fissures, having their rectums "stretched out," or becoming incontinent and having to wear adult diapers. In fact, the opposite is true quite frequently—people who practice safe, gradual, pleasurable anal sex have rectums that are as healthy as, and possibly healthier than those of people who don't have anal sex. Although it sounds surprising at first, the fact is that if you learn to exercise and tone your pelvic and sphincter muscles and regularly relax them during penetration, you are improving those muscles. The more you pay attention to your anus and rectum, the less alienated and anxious you will feel about it. The more you experience anal pleasure, the less likely your anus and rectum will be a source of tension—and tension is a leading cause of anal health problems. People who have more awareness of anal muscles and practice relaxing them are less likely to have recurring anal tension, difficult bowel movements, or problems like straining.

Your rectum and anal canal are used to expelling feces, not being penetrated by fingers or penises. Like everything else new, anal sex takes some getting used to. Right after having penetrative anal sex, you may feel like you need to have a bowel movement. In some cases, you do, and you should sit yourself on the toilet. In other cases, your rectum is simply adjusting to the experience of anal penetration; remember that the contractions of anal muscles experienced during anal sex and during orgasm are similar to the contractions of those muscles during a bowel movement. If you feel like you have to go to the bathroom, by all means, go. You may find that it was a false alarm; if you do have a bowel movement, you may also have a little irritation, soreness, and/or diarrhea or loose stool. When feces come down the anal canal they can mix with lube, making things a little runny. Some women feel minor bladder irritation and burning during urination after anal sex. All of this is temporary, and your urination and bowel movements should quickly return to normal. If problems persist or you have pain, extreme irritation, or bleeding, see a doctor.

In general, if you want to take care of your anus and rectum, make sure you do the following: eat enough fiber-rich foods; practice good hygiene habits; do not strain to have bowel movements; get enough exercise; and manage and reduce the general stress in your life. If you have anal penetration when it is uncomfortable or painful, it can lead to more muscle tension and damage to the delicate tissue of the anal and rectal walls.

Anal Ailments

Several factors contribute to the majority of all ailments of the anus and rectum: a lack of fiber and other deficiencies in your diet; chronic anal, rectal, and intestinal muscle tension; and general stress and tension. Safe, responsible anal sex in and of itself does not cause problems; however, sexual activity can exacerbate existing conditions. If you are experiencing recurrent constipation, diarrhea, itching, burning, irritation, pain, or bleeding in the anus or rectum or during bowel movements, you should see a doctor. Problems like constipation, intestinal disorders, hemorrhoids, anal fissures, or blood clots can usually be easily diagnosed and treated; however, if they are left untreated, they can lead to more serious complications and health problems.

Anal Sex and STDs

It is important for women to have knowledge about our bodies, including our vaginas, clitorises, breasts, and rectums. *You* are your best source of information; you know your body and its uniqueness better than anyone else. When you experience anything unusual—including rashes or sores, persistent itching, irritation, abdominal or pelvic pain, burning or pain during urination, any unusual discharge, irregular bleeding or cramping, or discomfort or pain during sex—you should see a gynecologist or other physician promptly. In many cases, you may have a simple, easily curable infection, but you could also have a sexually transmitted disease (STD). *For many women, STDs may occur without any symptoms at all*, so the only way they can be detected is through medical exams and laboratory tests. Therefore, all sexually active women should have checkups, pelvic exams, and pap smears on a yearly basis.

It is equally important to find a gynecologist or other physician you respect, trust, and feel comfortable talking to about your sexual health and practices. I've been to gynecologists who assume I'm heterosexual and ask me the requisite "What form of birth control do you use?" I've been to others who don't ask me anything about my sexual practices, partners, or concerns. Your gynecological visit is no time to play "Don't Ask, Don't Tell." If they don't ask, it's your responsibility to tell. While a regular exam at the gynecologist should include a pelvic exam, pap smear, breast exam, and rectal exam, many doctors do not perform rectal exams unless patients specifically present rectal symptoms. If you regularly engage in anal sex of any kind, you should inform your doctor, be frank about your practices, and request a rectal exam, even if you feel fine.

Sexually transmitted diseases can be rectal as well as vaginal. If you are diagnosed with an STD after a vaginal

Anal Sex Practices and Safer Sex

NOT SAFE: Unprotected rimming, unprotected anal finger-fucking, sharing anal sex toys without cleaning and disinfection or using a new condom; penis-rectum intercourse without a condom.

SAFER: Anal masturbation; rimming with a latex barrier; finger-fucking with a latex glove; cleaning, disinfecting, and using condoms with all sex toys; penis-rectum intercourse with a condom and withdrawal; fisting with a latex barrier; spanking or whipping that does not break the skin or draw blood.

exam and didn't have a rectal exam, you should return for a rectal exam. Because of the close proximity of our vaginas to our anuses, it is easy for women to spread infections from one orifice to the other. And if you had unprotected vaginal *and* anal sex, then the STD virus is likely to be living in both places; better to be safe than sorry. Most STDs can be treated and cured fairly easily with antibiotics if they are caught in their early stages. Untreated STDs can lead to more serious complications, including sterility, cancer, and, in some cases, death. So, please, take care of yourself.

Here are some of the most common STDs in America, their symptoms, and their treatments. I specifically discuss STDs that can be transmitted through anal sex and how the STDs affect your anus and rectum, since this book is primarily concerned with anal sex and health. Again, most women who contract an STD never exhibit symptoms until their condition becomes serious. You shouldn't attempt to self-diagnose an STD; use the following information as a guideline rather than a substitute for regular visits to the doctor.[1]

Anal Warts

Anal warts (like genital warts) are spread when your anal area comes into contact with the affected area of an infected partner. Anal warts begin as small pink bumps around the anus and in the anal canal; they tend to spread rapidly, forming clumps of bumps that may be itchy or painful if they are irritated. Their incubation period is usually one to six months. Anal warts are treated by removing them from the skin by applying chemicals to them (usually acids), burning them with an electric needle (electrocautery), or freezing them with liquid nitrogen (cryotherapy).[2] Even after visible warts are removed, the virus that causes them—the human papillomavirus

(HPV)—can remain in your body, and the anal warts can recur. You can also spread warts from your anus to your vagina and vice versa—another reason for regular rectal exams. If you have anal warts, you should also be checked for vaginal warts. Women diagnosed with anal warts should have regular exams even after they are removed to monitor recurrences and prevent complications.

Hepatitis

Hepatitis is an inflammation of the liver that has several different strains; I am going to address hepatitis A and hepatitis B because they are the most common and the most relevant to anal sex and health. The hepatitis A virus

---

Protecting Yourself

- Get tested for HIV and STDs regularly, especially if you have unprotected anal sex with partners.
- Always use condoms, dental dams, latex gloves, and water-based lubricants for all anal activities.
- Learn how to use condoms properly (see chapter 4).
- For an extra measure of safety during penis-rectum inter-course, have your partner withdraw before ejaculation. Remember, semen from men who are HIV+ has a high concentration of the virus and is very infectious.
- Safe, slow, and gentle anal sex decreases the chances of trauma to anal/rectal tissue; keep in mind, however, that you may already have minute tears or sores in the rectal lining that you don't know about.
- If you and your partner are both HIV+, you should still practice safer sex to avoid being exposed to a different strain of the virus or transmitting opportunistic infections.

is found in the feces of an infected person, so it can be spread by unprotected anal penetration and especially unprotected oral-anal contact. The hepatitis B virus is found in all bodily fluids of an infected person, including semen, saliva, vaginal secretions, blood, feces, and sweat. People with hepatitis may experience a variety of symptoms, including low energy, loss of appetite, depression, body aches, nausea, diarrhea, abdominal pain, rashes, swollen glands, fever, chills, dark urine, weight loss, and, if the condition has become serious, jaundice. Some people can be carriers of hepatitis and not have any symptoms; others can develop chronic, recurring hepatitis. People who are at risk of contracting hepatitis B can be vaccinated against the virus.

Genital Herpes

About 150 million people in the United States have been exposed to the herpes virus.[3] Genital herpes can be transmitted through sexual contact, including vaginal, oral, and anal sex; the herpes virus can also enter the body through mucous membranes or cuts in the skin. Within a week of exposure, people with herpes usually first experience a tingly or burning sensation in the genital area; then they develop bumps or blisters in the affected area, which can be itchy, sore, and/or painful. Women can also experience flulike symptoms, swollen glands or lymph nodes, a vaginal discharge or yeast infection, and painful urination. Initial sores usually heal in one to three weeks without treatment.

There is no cure for herpes, and symptoms can recur during outbreaks. These outbreaks can be brought on by stress, a compromised immune system, or prolonged exposure to the sun; they can last for up to three weeks. Although a person is most contagious during an outbreak, transmission of the virus can happen during nonactive periods as well (especially the two weeks after an outbreak) and with or without visible blisters or other symptoms. Sores can appear not only on but around the genitals, and condoms and dental dams will protect only the area they cover, so partners should limit their activities accordingly during outbreaks. In recent years, people with herpes have successfully used a drug called Zovirax™ (either ointment or pills) to control and treat symptoms.[4]

Rectal Gonorrhea

Rectal gonorrhea is transmitted exclusively through sexual contact. Symptoms appear within three to seven days of exposure and include soreness or burning during bowel movements and an anal discharge. Up to 80 percent of women who have gonorrhea have no symptoms, and this is even more true in cases of rectal gonorrhea than vaginal gonorrhea.[5] Rectal gonorrhea is treated with antibiotics, including penicillin, tetracycline, and ceftriaxone.

Chlamydia

The symptoms of chlamydia, which is transmitted through sexual contact, present one to three weeks after infection and are very similar to those of gonorrhea, including bowel movement discomfort, anal burning, soreness, and discharge; women may also experience swelling and soreness of the lymph nodes and rectal bleeding. Two-thirds of women, however, have no symptoms.[6] Chlamydia is also treated with antibiotics like doxycycline and azithromycin. Studies show that 45 percent of people with gonorrhea also have chlamydia, so people who've been diagnosed with one disease should definitely be tested for the other.[7]

Syphilis

Much less common today than in the past, syphilis is transmitted through vaginal, oral, and anal sex or through mucous membranes and cuts in the skin. It can have an incubation period of two to eight weeks. Ten to ninety days after exposure, people with syphilis experience the primary stage of the virus. A round ulcer (called a chancre) erupts in the affected area. The area in and around the chancre may ache or burn—or not. People may also have swollen lymph nodes. After the chancre hardens, heals, and disappears, the secondary stage begins. The secondary stage is marked by a general skin rash that may be itchy and painful. You may also experience fever, swollen glands, aching joints, headaches, nausea, and/or constipation. This stage is when people are most contagious. The third and fourth stages, latent and tertiary, are very serious and can be deadly if untreated. Syphilis is treated with antibiotics, usually penicillin, doxycycline, or tetracycline.

HIV and AIDS

Facts About Transmission

HIV, the virus that causes AIDS, is carried and transmitted through bodily fluids and most concentrated in blood, semen, menstrual blood, breast milk, and vaginal secretions. HIV is transmitted in several ways: through unprotected sexual contact with the bodily fluids of an infected person, by sharing needles with an infected person (through intravenous drug use), by receiving infected blood (through a transfusion), or from mother to baby via amniotic fluid, during delivery or breast-feeding. Current literature confirms that it's easier for women to get AIDS from men through sexual intercourse than vice versa.[8] This is because the tissue of the vagina is more susceptible than the tissue of the penis to trauma, tears, and minute sores, which provide infected semen a direct route to the bloodstream—and this is even more true of the tissue of the rectum. Also, semen has a higher viral load than vaginal fluid.

Women can transmit the virus to their women partners through unprotected oral and digital stimulation, especially if there are cuts or sores (which may or may not be visible) in their mouths or on their hands. They can also transmit the virus by sharing sex toys without using condoms or disinfecting them.

Finally, intravenous drug use is the riskiest route of all.

NOTES
1. For more information on STDs and anal sex, I recommend *Anal Pleasure and Health* by Jack Morin; *The American Medical Women's Association Guide to Sexuality*, edited by Roselyn Payne Epps and Susan Cobb Stewart; and *Your Sexual Health* by Dr. Jenny McClosky (San Francisco: Halo Books, 1993).
2. Morin, *Anal Pleasure*, 210.
3. Epps and Stewart, *Guide to Sexuality*, 140.
4. Epps and Stewart, *Guide to Sexuality*, 138–9.
5. McCloskey, *Your Sexual Health*, 164.
6. McCloskey, *Your Sexual Health*.
7. Epps and Stewart, *Guide to Sexuality*, 134.
8. Epps and Stewart, *Guide to Sexuality*, 152.

The Ultimate Frontier

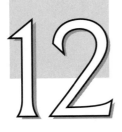

My goal for this book is to give women knowledge about their bodies, so we may all have safe, pleasurable anal erotic experiences. In my research, I have come across so many women who really enjoy anal sex—the unique physical sensations, the emotional intensity, the complex psychological dynamics. These same women took a major step in breaking their silence—a silence so wide-spread among all of us—to tell me that they love anal sex. Then they told me why they love to do it, how they love to do it, when they love do it, and with whom (or what) they love to do it. It felt great to finally hear other women's stories and not feel so alone with my own desires, fantasies, and experiences of anal sex. I hope *The Ultimate Guide to Anal Sex for Women* incites this kind of communication among its readers and that this important dialogue continues.

There are other books about anal sexuality in the works as this one goes to press, and I find that very exciting. There is so much more scientific, medical, and anecdotal research yet to be done on the subject. Just as each person's ass is unique, each person's particular take on anal sexuality is, too. We need more surveys, more stories, more guides, more information. Just think—the more information we have, the more anal sex we can have!

You obviously had the desire and curiosity to learn more about anal sexuality or you would never have picked up this book. If you've gotten this far, my desire is that you are now armed with information, resources, ideas, and some answers to your questions. Questions! People have so many questions about anal eroticism. I hope I have answered some important ones. I also hope that if you've got others, you'll ask them. Ask a friend, a lover, a health care professional, a sexologist, or one of the incredibly well-trained voices on the other end of the line at San Francisco Sex Information. The more I've brought up the subject of anal eroticism in my travels, the more people I've found who really want to talk about it. If we try not to censor ourselves, we just may learn something new—a simple how-to technique or even a secret hunger your lover never thought she could tell you.

Use this book with love, understanding, desire, and trust; ideally, it will reward you with some hot, sexy anal play. Remember that patience and practice make perfect. In my anal erotic experiences, I've felt sheer bliss, absolute surrender, indescribable rapture, and overwhelming pleasure—and I haven't gotten anywhere near perfect yet. In fact, I don't really want to. For me, the ultimate thrill is in the voyage.

Resources

Books

The American Medical Women's Association Guide to Sexuality by Roselyn Payne and Susan Cobb Stewart (New York: Dell Books, 1996). Although it may look like a conservative, straight-laced, dry medical guide, don't judge this book by its cover (or title); in fact, it's incredibly informative and has especially useful details on women's sexual health as well as STDs and how they affect both the vagina and the rectum.

Anal Pleasure and Health by Jack Morin (San Franicisco: Yes/Down There Press, 1986). As far as I am concerned, Jack Morin is the anal sex guru, and everyone should get a copy of this book; based on over six years of research, this latest of several revised editions is the most reliable source for information on anal sex. It also includes extensive work on psychological aspects of anal sexuality. A new edition is due in 1998.

The Complete Guide to Safer Sex edited by Ted McIlvenna (Fort Lee, NJ: Barricade Books, 1996). From The Institute for Advanced Study of Human Sexuality, this book is thorough, easy to read, sex-positive, and an invaluable source of information about sexuality and safer sex practices.

The Erotic Mind: Unlocking the Inner Sources of Sexual Passion and Fulfillment by Jack Morin (New York: HarperCollins, 1995). Another gem from Jack Morin, this book explores our most intense turn-ons and how they are often linked to our own life struggles.

The Essential AIDS Fact Book by Paul Harding Douglas and Laura Pinsky (New York: PocketBooks, 1996). One of the more recent books on the subject, this book offers clear, concise information on HIV and AIDS, including history, transmission, prevention, testing, health care, insurance, and legal matters.

The New Good Vibrations Guide to Sex by Cathy Winks and Anne Semans (San Francisco: Cleis Press, 1997). Subtitled *Tips and Techniques from America's Favorite Sex Toy Store*, this volume includes a wealth of information on sexual practices and techniques, anatomy, safer sex, and, of course, their specialty, sex toys. It also includes a super resource guide.

The Janus Report on Sexual Behavior by Samuel S. Janus and Cynthia L. Janus (New York: John Wiley & Sons, Inc.). Self-described as "the first broad-scale scientific national survey since Kinsey," this book analyzes the findings of a sex research project.

The Kinsey Institute New Report on Sex by June M. Reinisch, Ph.D., with Ruth Beasley, M.L.S. (New York: St. Martin's Press, 1990). Subtitled *What You Must Know to Be Sexually Literate*, this is the latest work based on the Kinsey-Roper survey done in 1989.

The Lesbian S/M Safety Manual, edited by Pat Califia (Los Angeles: Alyson Publications, 1988). Although this was compiled a decade ago, it has plenty of solid information on lesbian sexuality and S/M; just remember the AIDS information is outdated.

Sex for Dummies™ by Dr. Ruth K. Westheimer (Braintree, MA: IDG Books Worldwide, 1995). Dr. Ruth's guide to the basics of sexuality: anatomy, birth control, AIDS, romance, foreplay, after-play, masturbation, sexual health, and plenty of her therapeutic advice. You can also check out Dr. Ruth online at http://www.drruth.com.

Sex in America: A Definitive Survey by Robert T. Michael et al. (New York: Little, Brown and Company, 1994). The results of and commentary about a 1992 sex survey by social scientists.

Shared Intimacies: Women's Sexual Experiences by Lonnie Barbach and Linda Levine (New York: Anchor Press, 1980). A sample of interviews of American women about their sexual activities, styles, preferences, fantasies, and experiences. Frank, varied, and interesting.

Trust: The Hand Book (A Guide to the Sensual and Spiritual Art of Handballing) by Bert Herrman (San Franicisco: Alamo Square Press, 1991). The definitive guide to all aspects of handballing, or anal fist-ing, including preparation, techniques, safety, health, drug use, questions and answers, and the spiritual aspects of handballing.

The Woman's HIV Sourcebook: A Guide to Better Health and Well-Being by Patricia Kloser and Jane MacLean Craig (Dallas, TX: Taylor Publishing, 1994). An HIV/AIDS reference guide geared toward women, with information on transmission, prevention, testing, health care, relationships and family, and legal and financial concerns.

Your Sexual Health by Dr. Jenny McCloskey (San Francisco: Halo Books, 1993). An international best-seller, this book covers everything you need to know about sexual health, from anatomy to safer sex, with extensive information on STDs.

Publications

Anything that Moves
The quarterly magazine for the
uncompromising bisexual.
    2404 California Street #24
    San Francisco, CA 94115
    (415) 703-7977 x2

Bad Attitude
A magazine for lesbian and bisexual
women focused on erotica and S/M.
    P.O. Box 390110
    Cambridge, MA 02139

The Black Book
The best directory there is of sex-
positive services and organizations in
the U.S. and Canada.
    P.O. Box 31155
    San Francisco, CA 94131-0155
    (415) 431-0171
    (800) 818-8823
    http://www.queernet.org/BlackBooks
    BlackB@queernet.org

Black Sheets
A "kinky, queer, intelligent, irreverant"
zine of sex and pop culture.
    P.O. Box 31155
    San Francisco, CA 94131-0155
    (415) 431-0171
    (800) 818-8823
    http://www.queernet.org/BlackBooks
    BlackB@ios.com

Cuir Underground
A San Francisco based bimonthly
magazine for the pansexual kink
communities—people of all genders and
sexual orientations who enjoy S/M,
leather, fetishes, genderfuck, and other
forms of radical sexuality.
    3288 21st Street, #19-L
    San Francisco, CA 94110
    (415) 487-7622
    http://www.black-rose.com/cuiru.html
    cuirpaper@aol.com, curu@black-
    rose.com

EIDOS
Grassroots sex newspaper for "free-
thinking consenting adults of all eroto-
sexual persuasions."
    P.O. Box 96
    Boston, MA 02137-0096
    (617) 262-0096
    (800) 4UEIDOS
    eidos4sex@pipeline.com

Paramour
Magazine of literary and artistic erotica.
    P.O. Box 949
    Cambridge, MA 02140-0008
    (617) 499-0069
    http://www2.xensei.com/paramour/
    paramour@xensei.com

Shopping Guide

Sandmutopian Guardian
Practical, factual, pansexual guide to a
variety of S/M practices, written by the
people who do them.
    c/o Utopian Network
    P.O. Box 1146
    New York, NY 10156
    (516) 842-1711
    http://www/catalog.com/utopian
    siradam@ix.netcom.com

Trust, The Handballing Newsletter
    Alamo Square Distributors
    P.O. Box 14543
    San Francisco, CA 94114
    (415) 863-7410

Adam and Eve
Mail-order catalog of toys, videos, and
lingerie.
    P.O. Box 200
    Carrboro, NC 27510
    (919) 644-1212
    (800) 274-0333
    http://www.aeonline.com

Ambiance, The Store for Lovers
Retail stores offering toys, books, and
lingerie.
    Colonial Shopping Center
    7537 Mentor Ave.
    Mentor, OH 44060
    (216) 942-4669

    4745 Great Northern Blvd.
    North Olmstead, OH 44070
    (216) 779-4100

    6879 W. 130th St.
    Parma Heights, OH 44130
    (216) 885-2001

    20144 Van Aken Blvd.
    Shaker Heights, OH 44122
    (216) 751-2003

Arthur Hamilton
Mail-order catalog specializing in enema
equipment.
    P.O. Box 180145
    Richmond Hill, NY 11418
    (718) 441-6066

Ask Isadora
Audiotapes of world-renowned sex
advice columnist Isadora Alman.
   Isadora Alman
   3145 Geary Blvd. #153
   San Francisco, CA 94118
   (415) 386-5090
   http://www.askisadora.com
   isadora@sfbayguardian.com

A Woman's Touch
A feminist retail store of toys, books,
and safer sex supplies.
   600 Williamson Street
   Madison, WI 53703
   (608) 250-1928
   wmstouch@aol.com

Behind Closed Doors
Mail-order catalog of toys, books, and
videos for women.
   P.O. Box 93
   Woonsocket, RI 02895-0779
   (800) 350-3314
   ccondon@tiac.net

Betty Dodson, PhD.
Self-loving books and videos.
   P.O. Box 1933
   Murray Hill Station
   New York, NY 10156

Blowfish
Mail-order catalog of toys, books, and
videos.
   2261 Market Street #284
   San Francisco, CA 94114-1600
   (415) 285-6064
   (800) 325-2569
   http://www.blowfish.com
   info@blowfish.com

Chase Products
Medical equipment and supplies; good
place for enema accessories.
   P.O. Box 1014
   Novi, MI 48376-1014
   (248) 348-8191
   chase@wwnet.com

Come Again Erotic Emporium
Store and mail-order catalog of toys,
books, and lingerie.
   353 E. 53rd Street
   New York, NY 10022
   (212) 308-9394

Come As You Are
   701 Queen Street West
   Toronto, Ontario
   Canada M6J 1E6
   (416) 504-7934

Condomania
Retail stores and mail-order catalog of
condoms and safer sex supplies.

7306 Melrose Avenue
Los Angeles, CA
(213) 933-7865

351 Bleecker Street
New York, NY
(212) 691-9442
http://www.condomania.com

Crimson Phoenix
Retail store of books, toys, and
novelties.

1876 SW 5th Avenue
Portland, OR 97201
(503) 228-0129

The Crypt
Retail store of toys, videos, and fetish
wear.

1712 E. Broadway
Long Beach, CA 90802
(310) 983-6560

Diversified Services
Mail-order catalog for toys and nonfic-
tion D/S publications.

P.O. Box 35737
Brighton, MA 02135
(617) 787-7426
john-warren@msn.com

Dressing for Pleasure
Retail store and mail-order catalog
of toys and clothing, specializing in
fetish wear.

P.O. Box 43079
Upper Montclair, NJ 07043
(201) 746-4200 mail-order
(201) 746-5466 store

Eve's Garden
Woman-oriented store and catalog of
toys, books, and videos.

119 W. 57th Street #420
New York, NY 10019-2383
(212) 757-8651
(800) 848-3837
http://www.evesgarden.com
evesgarden@focusint.com

Fantasy Unlimited
Retail store of toys, books, magazines,
and fetish wear.

102 Pike Street
Seattle, WA 98101
(206) 682-0167

Focus International
Mail-order catalog of sexual health education pamphlets and videos.

1160 E. Jericho Turnpike
Huntington, NY 11743
(516) 549-5320
http://www.sex-help.com/

Forbidden Fruit
Retail store of condoms, lubes, toys, and
fetish wear.
   512 Neches
   Austin, TX 78701
   (512) 487-8358

Good Vibrations
Retail stores and mail-order catalog of
books, toys, and videos.
   Store:
   1210 Valencia Street
   San Francisco, CA 94110
   (415) 974-8980

   Store:
   2504 San Pablo Avenue
   Berkeley, CA 94702
   (510) 841-8987

   Mail-order:
   938 Howard Street #101
   San Francisco, CA 94103
   (415) 974-8990
   (800) 289-8423
   http://www.goodvibes.com
   goodvibe@well.com

Grand Opening
Retail stores and mail-order catalog of
books, toys, and videos.
   318 Harvard Street #32
   Arcade Building, Coolidge Corner
   Brookline, MA 02146
   (617) 731-2626
   http://www.grandopening.com
   grando@tiac.net

Intimate Treasures
Mail-order catalog of toys and videos;
subscriptions to "catalog of catalogs."
   P.O. Box 77902
   San Francisco, CA 94107
   (415) 863-5002
   http://www.intimatetreasures.com

It's My Pleasure
Feminist retail store of toys, books, and
videos.
   4258 SE Hawthorne Blvd.
   Portland, OR 97215
   (503) 236-0505

Lovecraft
Retail stores and on-line catalog of toys,
books, videos, and lingerie.
   63 Yorkville Ave.
   Toronto, Ontario
   Canada M5R 1B7
   (416) 923-7331

   2200 Dundas Street East
   Mississauga, Ontario
   Canada L4X 2V3
   (905) 276-5772
   http://www.regesex.com/lovecraft

Loveseason
Retail stores and mail-order catalog of
toys, videos, books, and lingerie.
   4001 198th Street SW #7
   Lynnwood, WA 98036
   (206) 775-4502
   (800) 500-8843

   12001 NE 12th Street
   Bellvue, WA 98005

Passion Flower
Retail store of toys, books, videos, and
lingerie.
   4 Yosemite Ave.
   Oakland, CA 94611
   (510) 601-7750
   passion@passionflwr.com

Pleasure Chest
Retail store and catalog of toys and
clothing.
   7733 Santa Monica Blvd.
   West Hollywood, CA 90046
   (213) 650-1022 store
   (800) 75-DILDO mail-order
   http://www.thepleasurechest.com

Romantasy
Retail store and catalog of toys, books,
and lingerie.
   2191 Market Street
   San Francisco, CA 94114
   (415) 487-9909
   (800) 922-2281
   info@romantasy.com
   http://www.romantasy.com

Rubber Tree
Retail store for safer sex supplies.
   4426 Burke Avenue North
   Seattle, WA 98103
   (206) 663-4750

Sin
Retail store and catalog of fetish wear.
   1512 11th Street
   Seattle, WA 98122
   (206) 621-0397
   (800) 315-7466
   http://www.sin-inc.com
   sin@aa.net

Spartacus Leathers
   300 SW 12th Avenue
   Portland, OR
   (503) 224-2604

The Stockroom
Retail store and catalog of toys and
clothing.
   4649 1/2 Russell Avenue
   Los Angeles, CA 90027
   (213) 666-2121
   (800) 755-TOYS
   http://www.stockroom.com
   info@stockroom.com

Stormy Leather
Retail store of toys and clothing, specializing in leather and fetish wear.
   1158 Howard Street
   San Francisco, CA 94103
   (415) 626-1672
   http://www.stormyleather.com
   info@www.stormyleather.com

Sex Information Resources

Toys in Babeland
Retail store and catalog of toys, books, and videos.
> 711 E. Pike Street
> Seattle, WA 98122
> (206) 328-2914
> (800) 658-9119
> Babeland@aol.com
> letters@babeland.com
> http://www.babeland.com

Voyages Catalog Group
Mail-order catalog of toys, videos, and other adult catalogs.
> P.O. Box 78550
> San Francisco, CA 94107
> (415) 863-4822
> http://www.voyages.com

Xandria Collection
Mail-order catalogs of toys, books, and videos.
> 165 Valley Drive
> Brisbane, CA 94005
> (415) 468-3812
> (800) 242-2823

American Social Health Association
A nongovernmental organization devoted to the prevention and control of all sexually transmitted diseases.
> P.O. Box 13827
> Research Triangle Park, NC 27709
> (919) 361-8400

Centers for Disease Control National AIDS Clearinghouse
> P.O. Box 6003
> Rockville, MD 20849-6003
> (800) 342-AIDS
> http://www.cdcnac.com

E-SIG
A special-interest group for lovers of enema erotica. E-SIG hosts an informative Web site on enema information.
> c/o AMTI
> P.O. Box 64307
> Virginia Beach, VA 23467-4307
> (757) 495-2564 fax
> http://204.141.230.178/esig-www/pages/info01.htm#Index
> WaterLuv@etzine.com

Human Awareness Institute
An organization that produces workshops on love, intimacy, and sexuality.
> 1730 S. Amphlett Blvd., Suite 225
> San Mateo, CA 94402-2712
> (415) 571-5524, (800) 800-4117
> http://www.hai.org
> office@hai.org

Institute for the Advanced Study of
Human Sexuality (IASHS)
School with a postgraduate degree pro-
gram in human sexuality studies. IASHS
also produces educational pamphlets,
books, and videos and safer sex supply kits.
    1523 Franklin Street
    San Francisco, CA 94109
    The Institute Sex Information
    Network: (900) CAN-HEAR ($2/min.)

The Kinsey Institute
    Indiana University
    Bloomington, IN 47405
    http://www.indiana.edu/~kinsey/

Los Angeles Sex Education Resources
    (213) 486-4421

National STD Hotline
    (800) 227-8922

Planned Parenthood
    (800) 230-PLAN
    http://www.ppfa.org

San Francisco Sex Information
    P.O. Box 881254
    San Francisco, CA 94188-1254
    (415) 989-7374
    http://www.sfsi.org

The Sex Institute
    513 Broadway
    New York, NY 10012
    (212) 674-7111
    SexQuest: http://www.sexquest.com
    rjnoon@sexquest.com

Sexuality Information and Education
Council of the U.S. (SIECUS)
A national, nonprofit advocacy
organization that develops, collects, and
disseminates information, promotes
comprehensive education about
sexuality, and advocates the rights of
individuals to make responsible sexual
choices.
    130 W. 42nd Street, Suite 350
    New York, NY 10036-7802
    (212) 819-9770
    http://www.siecus.org
    siecus@siecus.org

Society for Human Sexuality
A social and educational organization
devoted to the understanding and
expression of all safe and consensual
forms of human sexuality. Locally, SHS
serves the Seattle area, but anyone can
take advantage of their incredibly thorough Web site, which covers everything
having to do with sexuality: magazines,
books, videos, information lines, organizations, conferences, mail-order
resources, local resources in Seattle,
WA, and Portland, OR, plus links to
other sex-related Web sites.
    University of Washington
    SAO 141
    Box 352238
    Seattle, WA 98195
    (206) 526-5328
    http://weber.u.washington.edu/~sfpse

The Society for the Scientific Study of
Sexuality (SSSS)
An international organization dedicated
to the advancement of knowledge about
sexuality.
    P.O. Box 208
    Mount Vernon, IA 52314
    (319) 895-8407
    http://www.ssc.wisc.edu/ssss/

The Virgina Johnson Masters
Learning Center
The co-founder of the Masters and
Johnson Institute runs this center which
provides audiotapes, videos, seminars,
workshops, an informative Web site,
and other materials on sexuality,
intimacy, love, and relationships.
    10803 Olive Blvd., Suite 200
    St. Louis, MO 63141
    (314) 991-0341
    http://www.vjmlc.com
    drvjm@vjmlc.com

World Wide Web Resources

Alternate Sources
http://www.alternate.com
The only global CD-ROM, directory,
and Web site search engine for all the
alternate sexuality communities. They
also publish a directory.

Alt Sex
http://www.altsex.org
A Web site dedicated to BDSM, homo-
sexuality, bisexuality, polyamory, sexual
health, and transgender issues.

Alt Sex Anal Sex FAQs
http://www.halcyon.com/elf/altsex/anal-
sex.html

American Board of Sexology
http://www.indiana.edu/~kinsey/ASB/ne
whome.html

Charles Haynes's Radical Sex
http://www.fifth-
mountain.com/radical_sex
A directory of links to other radical sex
sites.

Coalition for Positive Sexuality (CPS)
http://www.positive.org
A quick-and-easy online tour through
the most important topics for teens who
are sexually active or thinking about
having sex.

Femme Productions
http://www.royalle.com
Run by Candida Royalle, Femme produces erotic videos from a woman's perspective, along with this informative Web site. Online catalog, interactive forums, and the "Ask Candida" advice column.

InstaTek Human Sexuality Site
http://www.instatek.com/sex/start.html
Information on bondage and discipline, S/M, BDSM resources, sexual activities, and sexual ethics.

IASHS Sexology NetLine
http://www.netaccess.on.ca/~sexorg/index.htm
A Web site dedicated to the advancement of knowledge of human sexuality. It includes information on sexual topics, questions and answers, a resource list, conferences and workshops, and other sexology links.

Queer Resources Directory
http://www.qrd.org
QRD has over 20,000 files and links about everything queer.

Sex, etc.
http://www.-rci.rutgers.edu/~sxetc
An online newsletter of information on sex, abstinence, contraception, AIDS, STDs, drugs, health, and more, produced by teens for teens.

Sexual Health InfoCenter
http://www.sexhealth.org/infocenter/info main.htm
A public service of Renaissance Discovery, this Web site has a guide to safer sex, STDs, lesbian/gay/bisexual issues, and sexual problems.

Index

A

adult bookstores, 48n, 56, 65
advice columns, 2
Ages of Lulu, The, 48n
AIDS, 11, 128-129; and anal sex, 3-4,
    18-19; and gay men, 4; and
    heterosexuals, 4; and lesbians, 4
Albert, Eric, 91, 101n
alcohol and drugs, 45-47, 92
American Medical Women's Association,
    35
*American Medical Women's Association
    Guide to Sexuality, The*, 36, 38n,
    129n
amniotic fluid, 128
amoeba, 33, 84
amyl-nitrite, 46
anal beads, 10, 50, 63
anal canal, 16, 21-30, 32-33, 67, 88
anal health, 4, 7, 11, 32-33, 121-129
Anal Pleasure and Health, 5, 6, 14, 20n,
    38n, 129n
anal sex, defined, 8-9; etymology, 8;
    and gay men. 2. 4, 14, 16-17,
    103-104; in film, 6; and heterosexual
    men, 17; and heterosexual women,
    17, 103-104; and lesbians, 103-104;
    media representations, 6-7; myths,
    2-4, 8-9, 13-20, 41-43, 102-104,
    112, 120; in porn, 6,98;
    preparations, 16, 31-37, 77-78,
    87-88, 107-108; psychological
    aspects, 4, 8, 10, 130; research, 8-9;
    taboo 2-4, 8-9, 13-14, 19, 41-42, 113
anal sleeve, 50
anal warts, 124-125

analingus, 1, 10, 18, 51, 53, 81-85, 94
anatomy, 10; anorectal, 21-30; female,
    22, 28-29, 76; male, 29-30
antibiotics, 127-128
anus, 11, 16, 21-30, 51, 55, 75-76,
    79-80, 82, 121, 124
Aqua Lube, 57
"Ariel," 119n
"Ass Forward," 48n
AstroGlide, 56
Aveeno Shaving Gel™, 73
azithromycin, 127

B

baby oil, 59
bacteria, 22, 32-33, 35, 54, 59, 84,
    107-108
Bakos, Susan Crain, 18, 20n, 48n
balls, 100
bathing, 22, 33-34, 78
Beasley, Ruth, 20n, 38n
"Beauty: The Rites of Purification," 73n
Beauty's Release, 73n
Best American Erotica 1997, 101n
Best Lesbian Erotica 1998, 66n
Betadine, 31, 64
birth control, 7, 123
bladder, 22, 29, 121
Blank, Joani, 101n
bleach, 31, 64, 72
bleeding, 111, 122, 127
blood, 126
body modification, 113
bondage, 5, 15, 113, 115
bowel movement, 16, 23, 32-33, 68-69,
    72-73, 121-122

bowels, 16, 73; empty, 32, 67
Brame, Gloria, 119n
Brantley, Cynthia, 20n
breast exam, 123
breast-feeding, 128
breathing, 25-26, 78, 107
Bright, Susie, 17, 20n, 40m 48n, 101n
bulb syringe, 68-69
butt plug, 1, 10, 17, 50-51, 58-60,
    80, 93, 97, 115; cleaning, 31;
    harness, 59; size, 59-60, 93;
    vibrating, 50, 60
buttocks, 27, 79, 81, 87

C

Califia, Pat, 103, 108, 111n, 119n
"Calyx of Isis, The," 111n
ceftriaxone, 127
chancre, 128
child birth, 128
Chlamydia, 127
chucks, 108-109
clitoral stimulation, 25, 47-48, 60, 76-78,
    87-88, 95-96, 98, 100
clitoris, 22, 76, 82, 123
colitis, 73
colon, 33, 82, 105
colonic, see enema
Comfort, Dr. Alex, 3, 12n
Coming to Power, 119n
communication, 9-10, 40-46, 82, 86,
    89, 91-93, 110, 115, 130-131
Complete Guide to Safer Sex, The, 37,
    38n, 66n
Condomania, 65
condoms, 32, 51-55, 57, 61, 84-85,
    105-106, 125, 127; animal skin, 55;
    female, 52-53; "natural," 55;
    ribbed, 55; and sex toys, 31, 61, 63
consciousness-raising, 75

constipation, 33, 41, 122
Cooper, Dennis, 6
Craig, Jane MacLean, 38n
Crisco, 57, 59, 105
cross-dressing, 5, 15, 117-118
cryotherapy, 124
cunnilingus, 81-82, 84, 129
Current Diagnosis and Treatment in
    Gastroenterology, 38n

D

dental dam, 10, 51, 54, 57, 84-85, 125,
    127
desire, 10, 39-40, 42-44
Details, 20n, 38n
deviance, 13, 112
diarrhea, 33, 41, 69, 121-122
diet, 32, 107, 121-122
Different Loving, 119n
"Different Place, A," 38n
dildo, 1, 10, 43, 50-51, 53, 59, 61-62,
    78, 80, 93, 97-98, 116, 118;
    cleaning, 31; harness, 17, 62; jelly,
    61; nightstick, 50; realistic, 50, 61;
    silicone, 61; size, 93; vibrating, 50
discipline, 5, 113
Dodson, Betty, 76-77, 80n
dominance, 5, 112, 115
douching, 10, 67
Douglas, Paul Harding, 38n
doxycycline, 127-128
drug stores, 56, 69, 106

E

E. coli bacteria, 33
Eat Me, 84n, 119n
Elbow Grease, 57
electrocautery, 124
Embrace, 57
emotional safety, 43, 39-48, 90

enema, 10, 16, 33, 67-73, 82, 107-108, 111; bag, 68-69, 71; coffee, 72; equipment, 68, 72; eroticized, 67; high colonic, 67; shower attachment, 68; vodka, 72
Epps, Roselyn Payne, 38n, 129n
erogenous zone, 22
Eros Bodyglide, 57
erotica, 5-6; gay men, 7; lesbian, 6; literature, 11
Essential AIDS Fact Book, The, 38n
"Every Boy," 66n
expectations, 42-44

F

fantasy, 10, 42-44, 104
fear, 9-10, 41-42
feces, 16, 22-23, 32-33, 54, 82, 84, 121, 126
fellatio, 16-17
fiber, 32, 107, 121-122
finger cot, 51
fingernails, 31, 51, 78, 105
fissures, 122
fisting, 1, 10, 102-111
flagellation, 113
Fleet Ready-to-Use Enema™, 68, 72
fluid bonding, 34-37, 105
foreplay, 5, 33
ForPlay, 57
fountain syringe, 69
Friedman, Scott L., 38n

G

G-spot, 16, 28-30
gay men, 5; and AIDS, 3-4; and anal sex, 3-4, 57, 116; and fisting, 103-104; in pornography, 104
genderbending, 116
genderplay, 11, 116-118

genital herpes, 126-127
genital warts, 124-125
glans, 29
gloves, 31, 105; double, 54-55, 106; latex, 10, 31, 51, 54-55, 57, 76, 79, 84-85, 105-107, 125; opera length, 106;
golden showers, 15
gonorrhea, 127
Good Vibrations, 7
Grandes, Almudena, 46, 48n
Grendell, James H., 38n
group sex, 15
gynecological self-examination, 75
gynecologists, 7, 122-124

H

hair, 22, 73
handballing, see fisting
Hartley, Nina, 39, 42, 48n, 83, 84n, 101n
health care professionals, 131
hemorrhoids, 41, 122
hepatitis A, 33, 82, 84, 125-126
hepatitis B, 125-126
herpes virus, 126-127
Herotica: A Collection of Women's Erotic Fiction, 101n
Herrman, Bert, 28, 38n, 74n, 101n, 102-103, 105-108, 111n
Heterosexuality, 20n, 138n
high-risk, 3, 84
HIV, 3-4, 11, 18-19, 34-36, 51-52, 82, 84, 105-106, 125, 128-129
homophobia, 14
human papillomavirus (HPV), 124
hydrogen peroxide, 31, 64
hygiene, 10, 16, 22, 31-32, 82, 121

I

I-D, 57
Institute for Advanced Study of Human
    Sexuality, 37, 38n
intercourse, *see* penetration
intestinal disorders, 33, 122
intestinal virus, 32, 82, 84
IV-drug use, 128-129

J

Jaivin, Linda, 83, 84n, 113, 119n
Janus, Cynthia L., 20n
Janus, Samuel S., 20n
Janus Report on Sexual Behavior, The,
    20n
Johnson, Virginia E., 20n, 38n
Joy of Sex, The, 3, 6, 12n

K

Kegel exercises, 25-26, 63, 78, 107
Key, Dorian, 58, 66n
Kink: The Hidden Sex Lives of Americans,
    20n, 48n
Kinsey Institute New Report on Sex, The,
    20n, 36, 38n
kissing, 33
Kloser, Patricia, 38n
Kolodny, Robert E., 20n
KY Jelly, 57
KY Liquid, 56-57

L

labia, 22
latex, 10, 31-32, 34-37, 49-55, 84-85;
    allergy, 106-107; and lubricants, 56-57
laxatives, 72
Leather Daddy and the Femme, 119n
leather sex, 5, 7, 112-115
Leatherfolk, 119n
Leland, Elliot, 20n

Lesbian S/M Safety Manual, The, 6
lesbians, 6, 103-104
Little Birds, 101n
lubricants, 10, 35, 49, 55-59, 69, 76,
    79-80, 92, 104-105, 109, 121;
    and condoms, 53; and dental dams,
    51, 84; "liquidy," 56-57; oil-based,
    57-59, 104-106, 108; thick, 57;
    water-based, 56-57, 104, 125

M

Macho Sluts, 111n
mail-order catalogs, 48n, 56, 65, 71
Mainard, Chester, 7
"Mandra," 101n
massage, anal, 86; erotic, 5
Masters and Johnson, 32
Masters, William H., 20n, 38n
masturbation, 5, 10, 13, 30, 75-80
McClosky, Dr. Jenny, 129n
McIlvenna, Ted, 38n, 66n
McQuaid, Kenneth R., 38n
Michael, Robert T., 20n
Michaels, Magenta, 87, 101n
Miller, Sarah, 20n, 26, 38n
misinformation, 3-4
monogamy, 5, 34-35, 105
Morgan, Robert, 38n, 73, 101n, 103,
    111n
Morin, Jack, 5-6, 14, 20n, 38n, 129n
mouthwash, 84
mucosa, 73

N

naughtiness, 2, 19, 26, 113
negotiation, 115
nervous system, 23
Nestle, Joan, 24, 38n
New Good Vibrations Guide to Sex, The,
    16, 20n, 36, 38n, 66n

New Joy of Sex: A Gourmet Guide to Lovemaking for the Nineties, The, 3, 12n
Nin, Anaïs, 94, 101n
Nina Hartley's Guide to Anal Sex, 48n, 84n, 101n
nonmonogamy, 5, 34-37, 105
nonoxynol-9, 35-37, 106-107; and irritation of tissue, 35-36
Northwest AIDS Foundation, 66n

O

Old Testament, 14
oral sex, 5, 13; *see also* analingus, cunnilingus, fellatio
orgasm, 2, 16, 25, 63, 76

P

pain, 17-18; fear, 41; and pleasure, 5, 115
pap smear, 122-123
parasites, 33, 82, 84
patience, 10, 45, 93
PC muscles, 21-30; exercising, 23-26, 60, 121
pelvic exam, 122-123
penetration, anal, 10, 24-25, 29, 59-64, 79, 82, 86-111, 121; finger, 1, 18, 51, 88, 121; and G-spot, 29; hand, *see* fisting; insertive, 41-42, 61-62, 77, 86-90, 97; penis, 36-37, 51, 53-54, 59, 121, 125; and prostate, 29; receptive, 23, 28, 40-41, 46-47, 61, 77, 90-93; vaginal, 25, 29, 49, 51-52, 56, 101, 105, 128
penicillin, 127-128
penis, 1, 16, 29, 51, 53, 84, 87, 93, 97-98, 100; bulb, 20; base, 29
perineal muscles, 22-23, 29
perineum, 16

phone sex, 5
Pinsky, Laura, 38n
poppers, 46
porn magazines, 98, 104
porn videos, 43, 45, 78, 98, 104
positions, 92, 109; doggie-style, 83, 92, 98-99, 109; missionary, 95, 109; receptive partner on top, 92, 96-97; reverse spooning, 99-101; sixty-nine, 83; spooning, 99-101
povidone iodine, 31
power dynamics, 10, 47-48
pregnancy, 37, 52
presence, 45-47
Probe, 57
Probe Silky Light, 57
proctitis, 73
prostate gland, 16, 29-30, 61
pubic bone, 22, 29
pubococcygeus muscles *see* PC muscles

Q

Queen, Carol, 117, 119n

R

Réage, Pauline, 6, 114, 119n
Reality™ Female Condom, 52-53, 66n
rectal exam, 123-124
rectal tissue, 81, 51-52, 121, 125
rectosigmoidal junction, 27
rectum, 16, 21-30, 32-36, 55, 57, 67-68, 72-73, 78, 80, 98, 105-106, 110, 121-124; curves, 28, 61, 93, 99
Reinisch, June M., 20n, 38n
relationships, 34-35, 43
relaxation, 10, 33-34, 88, 90-91, 107, 109, 110; exercises, 76, 78
Religious Right, 17
Restricted Country, A, 38n
Rice, Anne, 70, 74n

rimming, see analingus,
role-playing, 5, 113, 115-118
romance, 5
Roquelaure, A.N., 74n

S

sacrum, 22, 29
sadomasochism (S/M), 5, 11, 15, 67,
   103, 112-115
safer sex, 3-4, 7, 10-11, 19, 31-32, 34-37,
   52-53, 84-85, 104-107, 122-129
saliva, 126
SAMOIS, 119n
San Francisco Sex Information, 36, 38n,
   131
Sapphistry: The Book of Lesbian Sexuality, 6
Saran Wrap, 84
Second Coming, The, 119n
Semans, Anne, 20n, 38n, 66n
semen, 36, 52, 55, 125-126, 129
seminal vesicle, 29
sensory deprivation, 113
Sensuous Magic, 119n
sex, education, 2, 4, 6-7, 14, 21; kinky,
   2, 15; manuals, 5-6, 21; research,
   2, 5, 11, 15, 130-131
Sex for Dummies™, 6, 38n
Sex for One, 80n
Sex in America: A Definitive Survey, 6,
   20n
Sex on Campus: The Naked Truth About
   the Real Sex Lives of College
   Students, 20n
sex toy cleaner, 31, 64
sex toy stores, 17, 48n, 56, 71, 109
sex toys, 10, 36, 49-66, 76; disinfecting,
   31-32, 64, 129; flared base, 50, 61,
   64, 76-77; safer sex, 36, 57, 59,
   129; smooth, 63-64; see also anal
   beads, butt plugs, dildos, vibrators

sexologists, 5-6, 131
sexual health, 7
sexual history, 34
sexual identity, 116, 118
sexual revolution, 102
sexually-transmitted disease (STD), 7, 11,
   18, 34-37, 41, 51, 82, 84, 122-129
shaving, 10, 73
"She Gets Her Ass Fucked Good," 101n
Shopping Guide, 65
shower bidet, 71
sigmoid colon, 22, 27, 29
silicone, 107
silver bullet, 71
sling, 109
Slippery Stuff, 57
SM 101, 119n
soap, antibacterial, 31
Society for Human Sexuality, 66n
Sodom, 14
sodomy laws, 14
speculum, 75
sphincter muscles, 21-30, 53, 77, 79,
   88-89, 120-121; external, 23, 27;
   internal, 23, 27; relaxation, 23, 33,
   59-60, 88, 120-121
STD see sexually-transmitted disease
Stewart, Susan Cobb, 38n, 129n
Story of O, The, 6, 119n
stress, 33, 121-122
submission, 5, 98, 112-115
surrender, 28, 41, 96
Susie Bright's Sexual State of the Union,
   20n
Susie Sexpert's Lesbian Sex World, 48n
sweat, 126
Sweeney, Robin, 119n
syphilis, 127-128

T

tailbone, 22, 27, 29
"Taking Him on a Sunday Afternoon,"
    101n
tantric sex, 5
testis, 29
tetracycline, 127-128
therapists, 7
thigh harness, 62
Thompson, Mark, 119n
tongue, 51, 81-85
top, 96, 106, 112
touching, 33-34
transgender, 5
transverse colon, 67
trust, 10, 47-48, 90
*Trust: The Hand Book (A Guide to the
    Sensual and Spiritual Art of
    Handballing*, 6, 38n, 74n, 101n,
    111n
Trust/The Handballing Newsletter,
    103-104
Try, 6
turkey baster, 72

U

urethra, 22, 29, 32
urethral sponge, 22, 28; *see also* G-spot
urinary tract infection, 32, 54
urination, painful, 121-122; after
    penetrative sex, 32-33, 121
uterus, 22

V

vagina, 22, 51, 55, 75-76, 82, 84, 87,
    100, 105-106, 122
vaginal discharge, 126
vaginal douche, 72
Vaseline, 59
vibrator, 1, 5, 10, 60-61, 78, 80, 87-88,
    93, 96, 110
volatile nitrites, 46
vulnerability, 1, 90

W

Web sites, 65
Westheimer, Dr. Ruth, 6, 37, 38n
Wet, 57
Wet Light, 57
White, Rose, 91, 101n
winking, 88
Winks, Cathy, 20n, 38n, 66n
Wiseman, Jay, 119n
Women's HIV Sourcebook, The, 36, 38n
women's movement, 75

Y

yeast infection, 32, 54, 126
Your Sexual Health, 129n

Z

Zovirax™, 127

About the Author

Tristan Taormino is series editor of the annual collection *Best Lesbian Erotica*, for which she has collaborated with guest editors Heather Lewis, Jewelle Gomez, and Jenifer Levin. She is co-editor of *A Girl's Guide To Taking Over the World: Writings from the Girl Zine Revolution*, (NY: St. Martin's Press, 1997) and *Ritual Sex* (NY: Rhinoceros Books, 1996) a collection of writing on sex, religion and spirituality. She is also publisher and editrix of the pansexual erotic magazine *Pucker Up*. Her writing appears in several publications and anthologies, including *The Femme Mystique, Heatwave: Women in Love and Lust, Sex Spoken Here, Chick-Lit 2*, and *Virgin Territory II*, as well as *On Our Backs, Sojourner, The Boston Phoenix, The Advocate, X-X-X Fruit, Venus Infers*, and *Blue Blood*. *The Advocate* named her one of the Best and Brightest Gay and Lesbian People Under 30. She lives in Brooklyn.

About the Illustrator

Fish is an illustrator and cartoonist whose credits include the zine *Brat Attack* and *The Topping Book* and *The Bottoming Book*. You can find her work at http://www.devildogcom.

THE ULTIMATE GUIDE TO ANAL SEX FOR WOMEN

Tristan Taormino

The Ultimate Guide Anal Sex for Women is the first self-help book on anal sex for women. Accurate how-to advice is combined with interesting, eye-catching sidebars— myths, excerpts of erotic stories, and colorful narratives illustrating sexual techniques. User-friendly, sexy, honest, and fun, *The Ultimate Guide to Anal Sex for Women* offers comprehensive information on all aspects of anal eroticism and anal health for all women—heterosexual, lesbian, and bisexual. This attractive, upbeat guide covers anatomy; taboos and myths; fantasy, gender-bending, and power play; latex, lube, and toys; relaxation exercises; analingus; penetration, including fisting; and anal health. Bibliography, resources, index.

$14.95   ISBN: 1-57344-028-0

THE NEW GOOD VIBRATIONS GUIDE TO SEX

Tips and Techniques from America's Favorite Sex-Toy Store

SECOND EDITION

Cathy Winks and Anne Semans

"The Best Sex Manual Ever Written" — *The Advocate*

Recommended by medical professionals and sex therapists. Ten years of selling sex toys in a women-owned vibrator store, Good Vibrations, have given authors Anne Semans and Cathy Winks a unique perspective on sex. After talking to thousands of men and women about sex, they've learned what real people enjoy doing in bed and what information can help anyone achieve a happier, more satisfying sex life. This invaluable bedside companion is the single best reference guide to expressing and sharing sexual pleasure ever published.

$21.95   ISBN: 1-57344-069-8

Great Sex Manuals!

Hot Erotic Reading!

Best Lesbian Erotica and *Best Gay Erotica* feature the steamiest, most thought-provoking lesbian and gay sex writing you'll find. Each year, guest judges selected from the queer literary world review the year's best erotica and choose the final collection, representing a wide range of styles and voices. Once again, we present the best in sexy, literate queer writing— sometimes dark, sometimes perverse, often strange and irreverent, frequently unconventional, but always compelling, provocative, and *hot*.

BEST LESBIAN EROTICA 1998
Tristan Taormino, Series Editor
Selected and introduced by Jenifer Levin
$14.95   ISBN: 1-57344-032-9

BEST LESBIAN EROTICA 1997
Edited by Tristan Taormino
Selected by Jewelle Gomez
$14.95   ISBN: 1-57344-065-5

BEST LESBIAN EROTICA 1996
Edited by Tristan Taormino
Selected by Heather Lewis
$12.95   ISBN: 1-57344-054-X

BEST GAY EROTICA 1998
Richard Labonté, Series Editor
Selected and introduced by Christopher Bram
$14.95   ISBN: 1-57344-031-0

BEST GAY EROTICA 1997
Edited by Richard Labonté
Selected and introduced by Douglas Sadownick
$14.95   ISBN: 1-57344-067-1

BEST GAY EROTICA 1996
Edited by Michael Ford
Selected and introduced by Scott Heim
$12.95   ISBN: 1-57344-052-3

Books from Cleis Press

SEX GUIDES

Good Sex: Real Stories from Real People,
second edition, by Julia Hutton.
ISBN: 1-57344-000-0   14.95 paper.

The New Good Vibrations Guide to Sex:
Tips and Techniques from America's
Favorite Sex Toy Store, second edition,
by Cathy Winks and Anne Semans.
ISBN: 1-57344-069-8   21.95 paper.

The Ultimate Guide to Anal Sex for Women
by Tristan Taormino.
ISBN: 1-57344-028-0   14.95 paper.

SEXUAL POLITICS

Forbidden Passages: Writings Banned in
Canada, introductions by Pat Califia and
Janine Fuller.
Lambda Literary Award Winner.
ISBN: 1-57344-019-1   14.95 paper.

Public Sex: The Culture of Radical Sex
by Pat Califia.
ISBN: 0-939416-89-1   12.95 paper.

Real Live Nude Girl: Chronicles of Sex-
Positive Culture by Carol Queen.
ISBN: 1-57344-073-6   14.95 paper.

Sex Work: Writings by Women in the Sex
Industry, edited by Frédérique Delacoste
and Priscilla Alexander.
ISBN: 0-939416-11-5   16.95 paper.

Susie Bright's Sexual Reality: A Virtual Sex
World Reader by Susie Bright.
ISBN: 0-939416-59-X   9.95 paper.

Susie Bright's Sexwise by Susie Bright.
ISBN: 1-57344-002-7   10.95 paper.

Susie Sexpert's Lesbian Sex World
by Susie Bright.
ISBN: 0-939416-35-2   9.95 paper.

DEBUT FICTION

Memory Mambo by Achy Obejas.
Lambda Literary Award Winner.
ISBN: 1-57344-017-5   12.95 paper.

We Came All The Way from Cuba So You
Could Dress Like This?: Stories
by Achy Obejas.
Lambda Literary Award Nominee.
ISBN: 0-939416-93-X   10.95 paper.

Seeing Dell by Carol Guess
ISBN: 1-57344-023-X   12.95 paper.

VAMPIRES & HORROR

Brothers of the Night: Gay Vampire Stories
edited by Michael Rowe and Thomas S.
Roche.
ISBN: 1-57344-025-6   14.95 paper.

Dark Angels: Lesbian Vampire Stories,
edited by Pam Keesey.
Lambda Literary Award Nominee.
ISBN 1-7344-014-0   10.95 paper.

Daughters of Darkness: Lesbian Vampire
Stories, edited by Pam Keesey.
ISBN: 0-939416-78-6   12.95 paper.

Vamps: An Illustrtated History of the
Femme Fatale by Pam Keesey.
ISBN: 1-57344-026-4   21.95 paper.

Sons of Darkness: Tales of Men, Blood and
Immortality, edited by Michael Rowe and
Thomas S. Roche.
Lambda Literary Award Nominee.
ISBN: 1-57344-059-0   12.95 paper.

Women Who Run with the Werewolves:
Tales of Blood, Lust and Metamorphosis,
edited by Pam Keesey.
Lambda Literary Award Nominee.
ISBN: 1-57344-057-4   12.95 paper.

EROTIC LITERATURE

Best Gay Erotica 1998, selected by
Christopher Bram, edited by Richard Labonté.
ISBN: 1-57344-031-0   14.95 paper.

Best Gay Erotica 1997, selected by Douglas
Sadownick, edited by Richard Labonté.
ISBN: 1-57344-067-1   14.95 paper.

Best Gay Erotica 1996, selected by Scott
Heim, edited by Michael Ford.
ISBN: 1-57344-052-3   12.95 paper.

Best Lesbian Erotica 1998, selected by
Jenifer Levin, edited by Tristan Taormino.
ISBN: 1-57344-032-9   14.95 paper.

Best Lesbian Erotica 1997, selected by
Jewelle Gomez, edited by Tristan Taormino.
ISBN: 1-57344-065-5   14.95 paper.

*Serious Pleasure: Lesbian Erotic Stories and
Poetry,* edited by the Sheba Collective.
ISBN: 0-939416-45-X   9.95 paper.

GENDER TRANSGRESSION

Body Alchemy: Transsexual Portraits
by Loren Cameron.
Lambda Literary Award Winner.
ISBN: 1-57344-062-0   24.95 paper.

Dagger: On Butch Women, edited by
Roxxie, Lily Burana, Linnea Due.
ISBN: 0-939416-82-4   14.95 paper.

*I Am My Own Woman: The Outlaw Life
of Charlotte von Mahlsdorf,*
translated by Jean Hollander.
ISBN: 1-57344-010-8   12.95 paper.

*PoMoSexuals: Challenging Assumptions
about Gender and Sexuality* edited by
Carol Queen and Lawrence Schimel.
Preface by Kate Bornstein.
ISBN: 1-57344-074-4   14.95 paper.

Sex Changes: The Politics of Transgenderism
by Pat Califia
ISBN: 1-57344-072-8   16.95 paper.

*Switch Hitters: Lesbians Write Gay Male Erotica
and Gay Men Write Lesbian Erotica,* edited by
Carol Queen and Lawrence Schimel.
ISBN: 1-57344-021-3   12.95 paper.

LESBIAN AND GAY STUDIES

*The Case of the Good-For-Nothing
Girlfriend* by Mabel Maney.
Lambda Literary Award Nominee.
ISBN: 0-939416-91-3   10.95 paper.

The Case of the Not-So-Nice Nurse
by Mabel Maney.
Lambda Literary Award Nominee.
ISBN: 0-939416-76-X   9.95 paper.

Nancy Clue and the Hardly Boys in *A
Ghost in the Closet* by Mabel Maney.
Lambda Literary Award Nominee.
ISBN: 1-57344-012-4   10.95 paper.

*Different Daughters:
A Book by Mothers of Lesbians,*
second edition, edited by Louise Rafkin.
ISBN: 1-57344-050-7   12.95 paper.

*Different Mothers:
Sons & Daughters of Lesbians Talk about
Their Lives,* edited by Louise Rafkin.
Lambda Literary Award Winner.
ISBN: 0-939416-41-7   9.95 paper.

A Lesbian Love Advisor by Celeste West.
ISBN: 0-939416-26-3   9.95 paper.

On the Rails: A Memoir,
second edition, by Linda Niemann.
Introduction by Leslie Marmon Silko.
ISBN: 1-57344-064-7   14.95 paper.

Queer Dog: Homo Pup Poetry,
edited by Gerry Gomez Pearlberg.
ISBN: 1-57344-071-X   12.95. paper.

WORLD LITERATURE

A Forbidden Passion by Cristina Peri Rossi.
ISBN: 0-939416-68-9   9.95 paper.

*Half a Revolution: Contemporary Fiction by
Russian Women,* edited by Masha Gessen.
ISBN 1-57344-006-X $12.95 paper.

*The Little School: Tales of Disappearance
and Survival in Argentina* by Alicia Partnoy.
ISBN: 0-939416-07-7   9.95 paper.

Peggy Deery: An Irish Family at War
by Nell McCafferty.
ISBN: 0-939416-39-5   9.95 paper.

THRILLERS & DYSTOPIAS

Another Love by Erzsébet Galgóczi.
ISBN: 0-939416-51-4   8.95 paper.

Dirty Weekend: A Novel of Revenge
by Helen Zahavi.
ISBN: 0-939416-85-9   10.95 paper.

Only Lawyers Dancing by Jan McKemmish.
ISBN: 0-939416-69-7   9.95 paper.

The Wall by Marlen Haushofer.
ISBN: 0-939416-54-9   9.95 paper.

POLITICS OF HEALTH

*The Absence of the Dead Is Their Way of
Appearing* by Mary Winfrey Trautmann.
ISBN: 0-939416-04-2   8.95 paper.

Don't: A Woman's Word by Elly Danica.
ISBN: 0-939416-22-0   8.95 paper

*Voices in the Night: Women Speaking
About Incest,* edited by Toni A.H.
McNaron and Yarrow Morgan.
ISBN: 0-939416-02-6   9.95 paper.

*With the Power of Each Breath: A Disabled
Women's Anthology,* edited by Susan
Browne, Debra Connors and Nanci Stern.
ISBN: 0-939416-06-9   10.95 paper.

WRITER'S REFERENCE

*Putting Out: The Essential Publishing
Resource Guide For Gay and Lesbian Writers,*
fourth edition, by Edisol W. Dotson.
ISBN: 1-57344-033-7   14.95 paper.

TRAVEL & COOKING

*Betty and Pansy's Severe Queer Review of
New York* by Betty Pearl and Pansy.
ISBN: 1-57344-070-1   10.95 paper.

*Betty and Pansy's Severe Queer Review of
San Francisco* by Betty Pearl and Pansy.
ISBN: 1-57344-056-6   10.95 paper.

Food for Life & Other Dish, edited by
Lawrence Schimel.
ISBN: 1-57344-061-2   14.95 paper.

COMIX

Dyke Strippers: Lesbian Cartoonists A to Z,
edited by Roz Warren.
ISBN: 1-57344-008-6   16.95 paper.

*The Night Audrey's Vibrator Spoke:
A Stonewall Riots Collection*
by Andrea Natalie.
Lambda Literary Award Nominee.
ISBN: 0-939416-64-6   8.95 paper.

*Revenge of Hothead Paisan: Homicidal
Lesbian Terrorist* by Diane DiMassa.
Lambda Literary Award Nominee.
ISBN: 1-57344-016-7   16.95 paper.

Since 1980, Cleis Press has published provocative, smart books—for girlfriends of all genders. Cleis Press books are easy to find at your favorite bookstore—or direct from us! We welcome your order and will ship your books as quickly as possible. Individual orders must be prepaid (U.S. dollars only). Please add 15% shipping. CA residents add 8.5% sales tax. MasterCard and Visa orders: include account number, exp. date, and signature.

How to Order
- **Phone:** 1-800-780-2279
  or (415) 575-4700
  Monday–Friday, 9 am–5 pm
  Pacific Standard Time
- **Fax:** (415) 575-4705
- **Mail: Cleis Press**
  P.O. Box 14684,
  San Francisco, California
  94114
- **E-mail:** Cleis@aol.com